"Fascinating collection of essays (Dispelled some common myths ar the way I think about my food. in feeling healthier. This book comes as no surprise from a great and very experienced dietitian, Joyce. From her years of helping my patients better their nutrition, with this book I'm glad to see Joyce can extend her expertise to help the world."

~**Rakesh C. Gupta**, M.D., F.A.C.P., F.C.C.P

"I read *Loving Healthy Living* with great pleasure. The foreword is well researched and informative. The book is successful in conveying important health and wellness information. The layout features the stories of people with various health issues and personal struggles followed by relevant, healthy, and delicious recipes. The result is an inspirational read in which you can share in this amazing journey with Joyce and Linda to choose to live a healthy, vibrant life."

~**C. Harfouch**, M.D.

"The energy within this book is a gift that will keep on giving, from its title, *Loving Healthy Living*, to its rich and easy to 'digest' content of yummy recipes, beautiful photos, images, and uplifting and inspirational messages. Joyce Hack radiates her love, passion, enthusiasm, and Joy for Life, and her generous, kind, loving, and thoughtful ideas and gifts bless the lives of many. I believe this book is one of her passion projects and thoughtful gifts. She is a JOYful, loving, and caring presence whose name reflects her pure Spirit—JOYce!"

~**Amie Grenier**
Life Flow Coach, Creator, Teacher, and Inspirational Speaker

"Joyce Hack and Linda McLeod have outdone themselves in creating this diverse masterpiece, *Loving Healthy Living*. Anyone facing health challenges or doubt can turn the pages in this book, find answers, and know that they are not alone. Each individual's life-changing journey in this book is inspiring, heartfelt, and educational. The recipes are a delightful bonus."

~**Rhonda Beyreis**,
Gourmet Raw Vegan Chef, Instructor & Nutrition Educator
Author, *Comfort Foods Vegan Style* (www.RAWndalicious.com)

Loving Healthy Living

Copyright ©2018 by Joyce Hack and Linda McLeod

All rights reserved.

AuthorSource
San Diego, California
www.authorsourcemedia.com

No part of this publication may be reproduced, stored in a retrieval system, or transmitted in any form or by any means—electronic, mechanical, photocopy, recording, or any other—without the prior permission of the author.

This book is not intended as a substitute for the medical advice of physicians. The intent of this book is to provide general information in regard to the subject matter covered. The reader should regularly consult a physician in matters relating to his/her health and particularly with respect to any symptoms that may require diagnosis or medical attention.

ISBN: 978-1-947939-06-6

Printed in the USA

LOVING HEALTHY LIVING

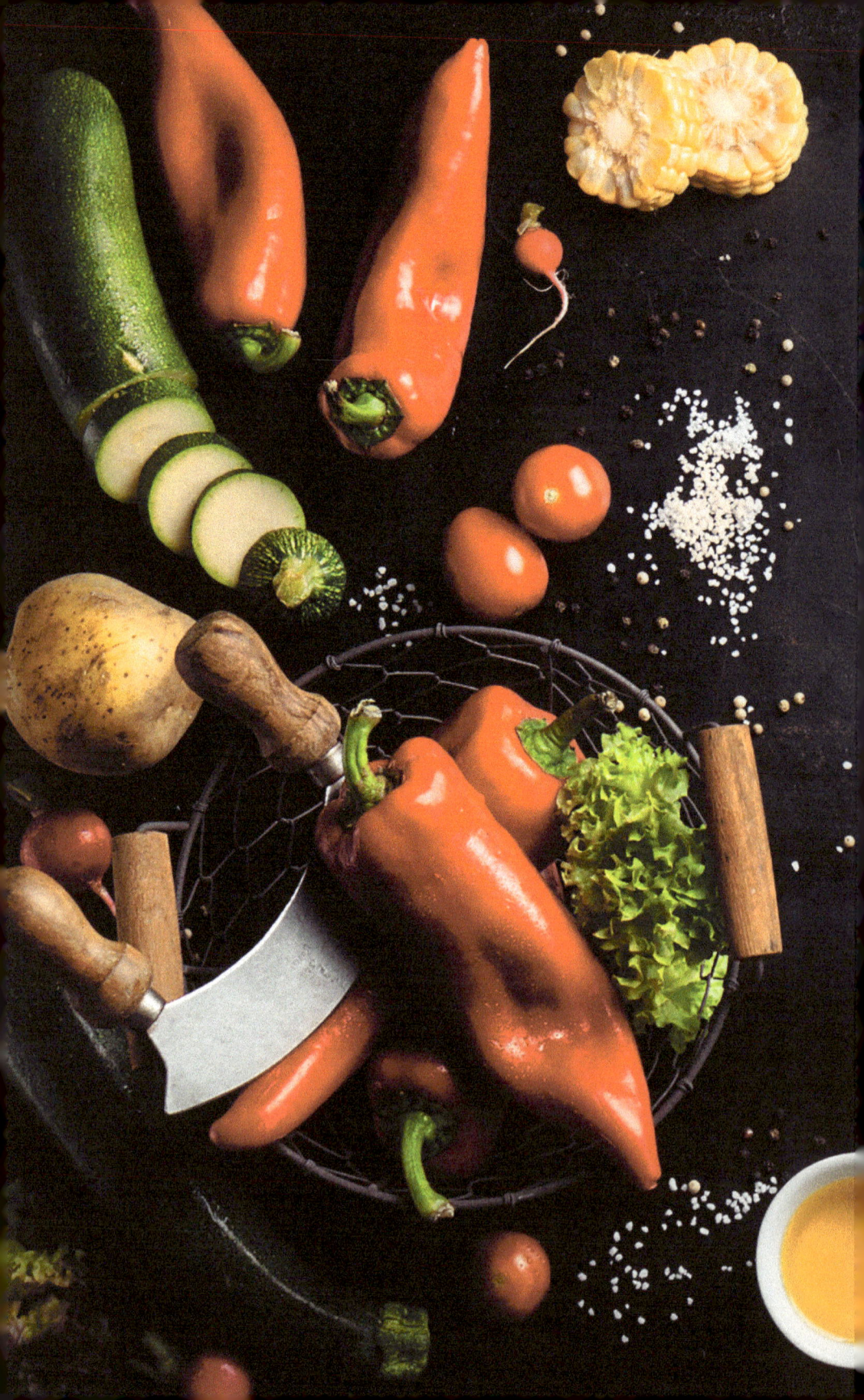

LOVING HEALTHY LIVING

30 LIFE-CHANGING STORIES THAT WILL INSPIRE YOU TO LIVE A MORE HEALTH-FILLED YOU!

Joyce Hack & Linda McLeod

DEDICATION

Joyce Hack

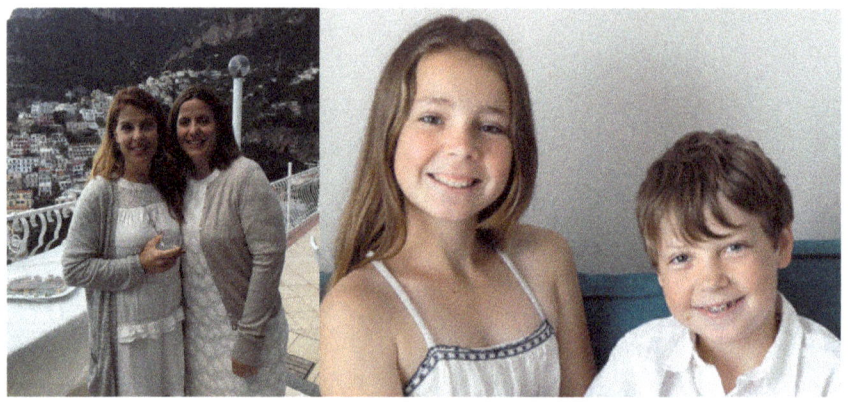

My daughters, Tiffany and Tamalyn, who taught me about love.

Life is precious, and it has to be lived for "love," the highest grandeur that life provides.

I take pride in seeing the wise women you are today, and I'm happy to share this glorious journey with you both.

My precious grandchildren, Madeline and Jack.

I delight in the children you were, now Madeline a teenager and Jack ten years old. You bring smiles and joy to my life every day.

A mother—and a grandmother—holds a child's hand for awhile, but their hearts forever.

DEDICATION

Linda McLeod

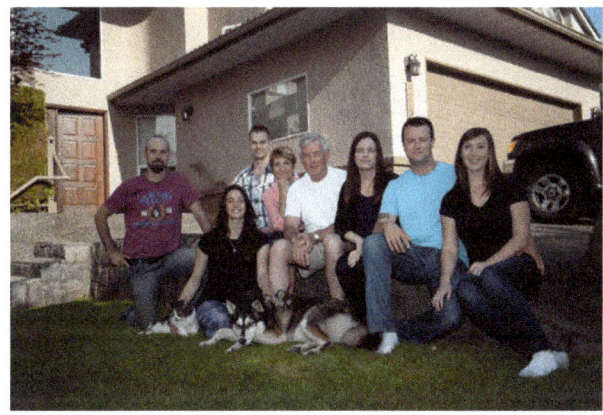

To the most important people in my life, who continue to be an example of how life should be lived in balance and to the fullest.

To Hugh, the love of my life, my husband, my best friend and life partner, you are my inspiration, and I cherish the life we have together. You mean everything to me, and you are the reason I live with gratitude every day. Thank you for all that you do to make our life together special.

To our blended family of five children—Colleen, Matthew, Aaron, Michael, and Jessica—who continue to share their lives with laughter, life stories, and a partnership that makes and keeps our lives strong. Each of you is so unique and wonderful in your own way, and the blessings you bring to our lives are amazing. I am proud of all your achievements and overflowing with gratitude for the love you contribute to my life and to our family.

TABLE OF CONTENTS

ACKNOWLEDGMENTS 13
FOREWORD 15
INTRODUCTION 17
THE POWER OF CHOICE 30
BATTLEFIELD OF THE MIND 34
Les Brown
A RETURN TO LOVE 38
Marianne Williamson
LOVE IS BEAUTIFUL 39
Joyce Hack
HEALTHY CHOICES HEALTHY LIFE 46
Linda McLeod
THE YUM STORY 52
Theresa Nicassio
SUGAR CAUSED MY ILLNESS 62
Stacey Morgenstern
MY BINGE EATING DISORDER WAS KILLING ME 66
Carey Peters
FROM FAT VEGAN TO SKINNY BITCH 72
Chef AJ
A TASTE OF SOUTHERN HOSPITALITY 80
Martha Green
A BRIGHT SIDE OF BAD HABITS 86
Chad Curtis
MY JOURNEY WITH GUT HEALTH 94
Tina Jordan Amoah
RAISING VOICES, LIFTING SPIRITS, CHANGING LIVES ... 100
Meg Zeleny

UNDERSTANDING FOOD SENSITIVITIES.............................106
Samantha Schmuck
I AM MY BEST FRIEND 112
Bertha Noble
NOURISHING MY BODY & SOUL WAS LIFE CHANGING..118
Nicole Jennifer Enns
CHANGE THE WORLD ONE PLATE AT A TIME 128
Brittany Johnson
LET FOOD BE THY MEDICINE..132
Hollie Ancharoff
I GOT MY LIFE BACK 138
Amber Anderson
A JOURNEY TO BETTER HEALTH 144
Kirsten Ault
NEW HABITS BETTER LIFE 150
Holly Kelsey
A NEW LEASE ON LIFE 156
Dan Ferrato
THE POWER OF FOOD 162
Dana Camera
FOR THE LOVE OF FOOD 168
Jessica Geist
HEALTH IS OUR MOST IMPORTANT ASSET 174
Lucie Woods
FOOD IS FOOD 180
Laura Stempky
DETERMINED TO BE HEALTHY & FIT 186
Donna Willon
CONSTANT PAIN TO GREAT HEALTH....................................192
Evelin Ledebuhr
THE NUT DOESN'T FALL FAR FROM THE TREE 198
Shawnya Michaels
REACHING MY IDEAL WEIGHT 204
Robin Moon

MY JOURNEY TO HOLISTIC HEALTH COACH 210
Charleen Cuellar
MAKE CHANGES NOW— DON'T WAIT 218
Peggy Heaton
LIFE IS A CANDLE 224
ABOUT THE AUTHOR: "TRAGEDY TO TRIUMPH" 225
Joyce Hack
ABOUT THE AUTHOR: "FROM HEALTH CHALLENGES
TO HEALTH COACHING" 228
Linda McLeod
RECIPE NAMES BY CO-AUTHOR 231

ACKNOWLEDGMENTS

With heartfelt thanks we express our deepest gratitude to our readers, contributors, and the incredible team who made this such a great book!

To you, our readers, for choosing this book and reading these amazing stories, and for your willingness to trust these life-changing stories and to be inspired to make life choices for a healthier you.

Thank you to each of the co-authors who were willing to share their incredible stories and healthy recipes with the world. Your stories inspire and awaken hope in our readers and encourage those who suffer from disease to take steps toward better health by allowing food to be the healer.

A very special thank you to Dr. Hans A. Diehl, DrHSc, MPH, CNS, FACN, Clinical Professor of Preventive Medicine, School of Medicine, Loma Linda University, Founder, CHIP and Lifestyle Medicine Institute, who has been our mentor and helped establish a high standard for the recipes in the book. His contributions were an invaluable addition, and we are grateful for his willingness to work with us. Dr. Diehl travels around the globe as a world-renowned health leader. Thank you, Dr. Diehl!

Mr. Les Brown is a world-renowned motivational speaker and author. His book is an inspiration and a great read. In his words, "It is not over until you win!" Mr. Brown, thank you for your contribution to our book.

We acknowledge and congratulate Carey Peters and Stacey Morgenstern, founders of Health Coach Institute, for their contribution in creating the world's most effective Health Coaching School. From their life-changing stories, they are now training and coaching a new generation of health and nutrition coaches who are changing the consciousness of the planet. To find out more, visit http://www.heathcoachinstitute.com.

Bshara Al-Sheikh, a young college student and IT guru, is on his way to accomplishing great things in life. Bshara, you have been amazing with bringing this book together. Thank you for contributing hours of your time to produce a complete manuscript for the publisher to work with. It has been a privilege and joy to have you on this exciting journey with us. Thank you for your continued support.

Joyce and Linda extend their deepest respect and gratitude for the team of qualified individuals who have contributed their time and expertise to publishing *Loving Healthy Living*. Thank you for believing in us and for your commitment to seeing this vision become a reality—one that will inspire others to choose a healthier path. Our publishing team includes Simon Presland, Ash Silva, Beth Lottig, and Tiffany Harelik. Thank you for giving your time, dedication, and energy to make this book a success.

If you wish to contact any of the authors, please send an email to Joyce Hack at joyinred@verizon.net or Linda McLeod at linda@healthhabits4life.com.

FOREWORD

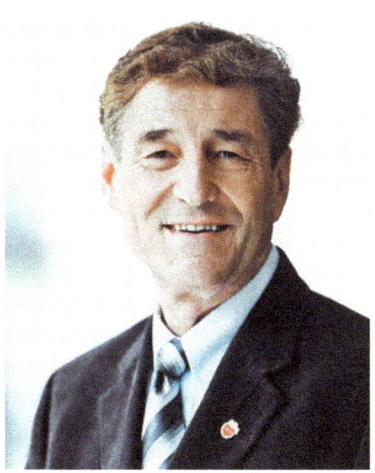

by Dr. Hans Diehl

Changing Habits, Changing Lives

It's a joy to write a few lines to welcome *Loving Healthy Living: 30 Life-changing Stories That Will Inspire You to Live a More Health-filled You!*

With many contributors, this compilation represents a dream come true for co-editors Joyce and Linda. They have both experienced transformations in their personal lives. Their success stories will inspire hope and an "I can" attitude. Undoubtedly, this will empower the reader to set and pursue new goals. Their success stories will also give credibility to their rewarding careers as health and wellness coaches. As such, they have clearly defined goals: helping others to achieve their best health and more fulfilling and balanced lives by providing guidance to change habits for lasting results.

The ladies know that by changing habits we can all change our lives. And the Greek philosopher Aristotle understood that more than 2,000 years ago. He wrote, "We are what we repeatedly do. Excellence is not an act but a habit." A habit is either the best of all servants or the worst of all masters. Habits either oil the machinery of our lives, helping us to glide through our days, or they rob us of energy and accomplishment.

More than ever we need to recognize the many options we have to influence and shape our lives and health outcomes. In this domain of lifestyle choices, nothing will easily take the pre-eminent role of our food choices. What we put at the end of our forks and spoons will either promote disease or health. A fork and spoon can be weapons of mass destruction or they can be instruments of health and healing.

More than 80,000 graduates from our Complete Health Improvement Program (CHIP) have validated the power of a more Optimal Diet coupled with a consistent, moderate exercise program. The clinical results have been published in more than forty scientific publications. An Optimal Diet focuses on eating more plant and unprocessed foods, while reducing the consumption of refined foods and foods of animal origin. Such a diet then would be low in salt, sugar, and fat and be almost devoid of cholesterol, yet high in nutritional density and fiber. When combined with a consistent exercise program, the clinical results of such a lifestyle have been shown to prevent, arrest, and facilitate the reversal of many of our modern killer diseases, such as heart disease, hypertension, diabetes, and obesity.

As *Loving Healthy Living* inspires you to try new foods and recipes, and to make new commitments to yourself and your loved ones, may your health soar and your life become a legacy witnessed by personal achievement and greatness through service.

"Everyone has the power for greatness, not for fame but greatness, because greatness is determined by service." ~Martin Luther King, Jr.

To your best health!

Hans Diehl, DrHSc, MPH, FACN

Clinical Professor of Preventive Medicine
School of Medicine, Loma Linda University
Founder of CHIP and Lifestyle Medicine Institute
Loma Linda, CA
www.chiphealth.com

INTRODUCTION

The Importance of an Optimal Diet

The accomplishments of modern medicine have been prodigious. We have seen the development of proton accelerators that can zap cancers, surgical robots that can be employed in performing coronary bypass surgeries, and advances in molecular biology and genetics that can open doors to amazing new worlds. Yet these advances in high-tech medicine have not altered the advances of our modern killer diseases.

Western Diseases Boom

Virtually unknown less than 100 years ago, coronary artery disease and cancers of the breast, prostate, colon, and lungs are now claiming every third and fourth American life, respectively. In spite of newer and refined forms of insulin and a plethora of bioengineered medications, the incidence rate of the common form of diabetes has gone up 300 percent over the last thirty years, with one in three children born today now developing diabetes before they die.

Concurrently, we have seen an enormous rise in the prevalence of excess weight, making it necessary for manufacturers to supersize everything from shirts to pants and from gurneys to coffins. At present, more than 35 percent of American adults are overweight, and another 36 percent are obese. By the year 2030 obesity is expected to increase to 50 percent.

The Myth of an Extra 30 Years

For years, we have cherished the belief that we are the world's healthiest society and that this new epidemic of so-called Western diseases was related to our extended life expectancy. After all, over the past 100 years, the life expectancy at birth has gone up twenty-nine years, from forty-nine to seventy-eight years of age. The justification of the steep rise in some of these chronic diseases was that our ancestors just didn't live long enough to die of these Western diseases of "old age."

However, the often-overlooked fact is that 100 years ago every sixth baby died before reaching the end of their first year of life, while today this number has been dramatically reduced thanks to improvements in public health, sanitation, and maternal health. It was the high mortality rate of newborns and children 100 years ago that greatly shortened the average life span. With this in mind, it's sad to see that sixty-five-year-old Americans today may have gained only six or seven years of life expectancy over their counterparts from years ago. Once people survived those early-childhood diseases, they had a reasonably good chance of living almost as long as today's seniors, and that in an era when very few medical interventions were available, and when less than 1 percent of the country's gross domestic product (GDP) was devoted to the cost of health care.

In contrast, we are now devoting 19 percent of our GDP, or over $3.5 trillion annually, to health care. This amounts to $10,600 for every man, woman, and child. It is obvious: The current system is unsustainable.

The Interventional Imperative

Ever since the estrogen dilemma, in which Premarin—then the number one prescription drug in America—was shown to cause more morbidity and death than benefit, other interventions, such as bypass surgery (400,000 per year at $150,000 each) and angioplasty (900,000 per year at $35,000 each), have been questioned.

Many physicians and patients don't know—or don't want to believe—that:

- Only 10 percent of heart attack patients have their life extended with bypass surgery.
- 38 to 46 percent of grafted vessels will have failed as bypasses within 12 to 18 months after surgery.
- 30 to 45 percent of angioplasty procedures are no longer functional within six months.

Surgical interventions for heart disease provide only limited sustainable clinical benefit, but they often generate 50 to 70 percent of a hospital's revenues. Pharmaceuticals, plagued by side effects, result in some 246,000 deaths per year, making prescription drugs the third-leading cause of death in America. No wonder many health policy analysts have felt that medical care has become largely a business-driven enterprise. They are increasingly aware of the tremendous pressures that pharmaceutical lobbies and massive marketing efforts exert on researchers, physicians, journal editors, government agencies, and the general public. They are also keenly aware of how, tragically, numerous procedures and medications are often accepted and widely used by many without adequate research to assess their effectiveness, safety, and long-term impact.

Medical Care versus Health Care

It is clear that the medical-industrial complex offers silver bullets that are all too readily picked up by health-care providers and consumers alike. Many mistakenly have been sold on the idea that medical care is synonymous with health care. Health, however, is largely a matter of personal responsibility that must be exercised within the limits of genetic endowment. With more than 80 percent of our well-being determined by lifestyle factors, medical care actually has relatively little impact on health.

Our health is largely a function of how people take responsibility for their own actions. Promoting health, therefore, has to do with addressing causes, not with symptomatic or palliative treatment, as helpful as that may be at the time. It has to do with education, motivation, and cultural transformation. Let's take a look at the nation's number one killer, heart disease, and its underlying disease process—atherosclerosis.

Atherosclerosis: The Silent Killer

We were born with clean, flexible arteries, and they should stay that way until we die of old age. The arteries of most Americans, however, are clogging up with cholesterol, fats, and calcium. This creates (1) unstable, soft plaques that can rupture and clog up suddenly causing most heart attacks and strokes and (2) stable, hard plaques that can gradually clog up, causing progressive angina and degenerative diseases.

This buildup of atherosclerotic plaques affects the circulatory system in different critical areas. While the clinical expressions of atherosclerosis may carry different disease names, the main underlying pathologic process is the same. It is atherosclerosis, and its low-grade inflammation reduces tissue oxygenation and leads to degenerative changes associated with angina pectoris, myocardial infarction (heart attack), intermittent claudication (peripheral vascular disease), gangrene, impotence, hypertension, cerebral infarction (stoke), senility, hearing loss, visual loss, and possibly some of the common adult cancers. In our society, this narrowing process commonly begins early in life and can be demonstrated in teenagers by way of autopsies.

With so many deaths taking place every year, one would expect more than a murmur of protest from the public, the press, or government agencies. Such a rash of killings by any other means would mobilize the county! Atherosclerosis is not a "natural" way to go. It's not the inevitable result of the aging process. Large populations in the world are unaffected by it. After World War II, the University of Tokyo's medical school had to import atherosclerosed coronary arteries from the United States to be able to show its medical students what was then killing every second American, since the disease at that time was so rare in Japan. With the importation of the rich Western diet, however, came the Western diseases. After only 20 years, Japan became totally "self-sufficient" in creating its own narrowed coronary arteries. They no longer had to import narrowed coronary arteries from Johns Hopkins University.

With close to 3,000 heart attacks a day in the United States, and with sudden death often being the first symptom of underlying coronary artery disease, what are the predisposing conditions? The first solid evidence came during World War II, when coronary disease rates in industrialized European countries dropped dramatically, with coronary arteries beginning to open up again, apparently in response to a simple, Spartan diet. Some 15 years later these atherosclerotic plaques, however, returned, as the typical affluent American lifestyle (with cigarettes, automobiles, and a rich diet) gradually became the hallmark of many European countries.

Research with monkeys has consistently demonstrated that atherosclerotic plaques can be created and promoted by feeding the animals a Western diet very high in fat and cholesterol. But they can also be reversed by removing these atherogenic dietary stimuli.

The Framingham Heart Study

Initiated in 1949, this monumental research conducted for almost 70 years now in Framingham, Massachusetts, led to the discovery of risk factors for heart disease and its underlying atherosclerotic disease process. This risk factor concept has become as important to heart disease as the germ concept has become to the infectious diseases.

Multimillion-dollar studies funded by the National Institutes of Health have shown that 63 to 80 percent of all major coronary events before age 65 could be prevented if Americans would lower their cholesterol (to less than 180) and their systolic blood pressure (to less than 125), and quit smoking. These simple changes in lifestyle would do more to improve the nation's health, productivity, and vitality than all hospitals, surgeries, and medical procedures combined.

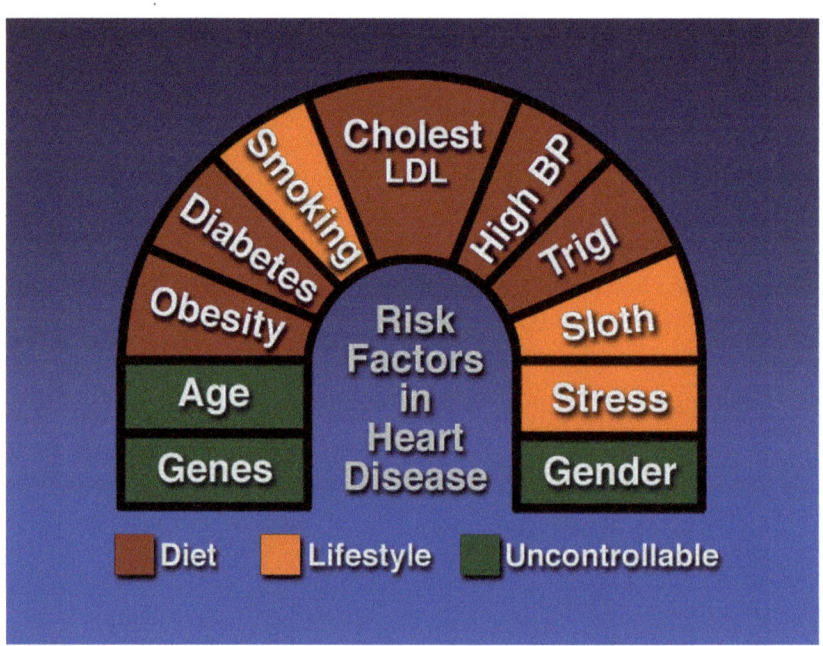

The Connection between GDP and Western Diseases

Examining the global distribution of Western diseases (with many prominently related to atherosclerosis), a strong economic gradient emerges: the higher the national income (Gross Domestic Product), the greater the prevalence of Western diseases (see Figure 2).

The China Study

The massive China Study, masterminded by T. Colin Campbell, PhD, of Cornell University, for instance, clearly showed two clusters of diseases in China. Populations surveyed near metropolitan centers displayed high rates of "diseases of affluence," such as coronary artery disease, stroke, hypertension, diabetes, osteoporosis, and cancer of the breast, prostate, lung, and blood. Rural populations, in contrast, suffered from "diseases of poverty," such as pneumonia and tuberculosis, digestive diseases, cancer of the stomach and liver, and infectious and parasitic diseases. While the diseases of affluence correlated closely with the level of economic development and abundance of processed foods, fast foods, and animal products high in fat and protein (eating meat in China has now become a status symbol and sign of prestige), the diseases of poverty were predominantly intertwined with poor sanitation, nutritional deficiencies, and poor food quality because of a lack of refrigeration.

The researchers concluded that, "Chinese counties with a more affluent lifestyle (a richer diet, more smoking, and less exercise) showed a clear shift from diseases of poverty to diseases of affluence." They added, "These diseases of affluence are not inevitable. Societies that can afford sanitation, refrigeration, and abundant food may yet conquer these diseases of affluence by simplifying their diet and by eating more foods-as-grown."

Changes in Diet Composition

Developing countries have to rely predominantly on foods-as-grown. They rely basically on corn and beans, potatoes and yams, wheat and rice, and plenty of fruits and vegetables. These inexpensive, yet nutritionally rich, plant foods provide more than enough protein, modest amounts of fat and sugar, and plenty of complex carbohydrates, the body's preferred and clean-burning fuel to meet energy requirements.

As the GDP increases, however, dietary sources change drastically (see Figure 2). Developing countries rely mostly on unrefined complex carbohydrate foods high in starch, which account for 70 percent of total calories (shown in green), with very few calories coming from fats, oils, sugars, and animal products. On the other hand, the diet of affluent countries is largely composed of fats and oils (36 percent of calories) and sugars (20 percent), shown in red and yellow, respectively. And their complex carbohydrates are usually refined, white flour products, such as pies, pastries, pastas, and pizzas, crowding out the nutritionally rich unrefined complex carbohydrates (now accounting for only 6 percent of total calories).

Diets incorporating foods-as-grown are naturally very low in fat, oil, grease, salt, and sugar, and usually very low in animal protein. Thus, they are almost devoid of cholesterol, saturated fat, and trans-fats (hydrogenated). Yet they are high in fiber and nutritional density.

As these countries become more affluent, however, foods turn into industrial products. Potatoes turn into Pringles, corn into Doritos, wheat into Zingers, oats into Oreos, and beans and grains turn into sirloin steaks. With food technology able to create new taste sensations on one hand, and with advertising able to create a mass market on the other, the diet composition undergoes a major overhaul—the largely unrefined complex carbohydrates become a minority player. In their stead, calorie-dense, processed foods—usually high in sugar (simple carbohydrates) and fats—as well as meats, sausages, eggs, and cheese high in fat, calories, and cholesterol become the dominant energy carriers.

Figure 2

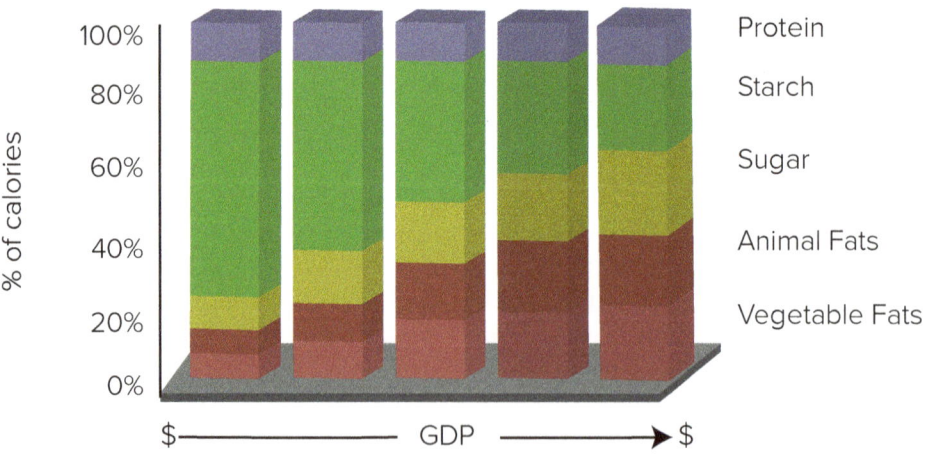

As the GDP increases from developing countries on the far left to the affluent countries on the far right, the dietary energy souces change drastically.

The Food Revolution

Food just isn't the same anymore. Some 100 years ago, the American diet consisted largely of foods-as-grown, coming mostly from local gardens and nearby farms. It was supplemented with a few staples from the general store and some meat from range-fed cattle. Our great-grandparents didn't have 50,000 slickly packaged, cleverly promoted products waiting at the local supermarket, or 95,000 fast-food restaurants spending billions of dollars advertising take-out service.

Families in those days sat at their own tables and ate their freshly cooked food and home-baked bread. But times and tastes and serving sizes have changed. Nowadays, many of us spend 60 percent of our food dollars "eating out." Our livestock is fattened in feed lots where a lack of exercise, antibiotics, and "growth enhancers" produce bigger cattle and juicier meat with about twice as much fat as range-fed cattle. Farm produce is processed, refined, concentrated, sugared, salted, and chemically engineered to produce taste sensations that are rich in calories but poor in nutritional value. Advertising and marketing have created a demand that produces big profits and big bodies.

Foods-as-grown are different. They are nutritionally balanced. They don't need nutrition labels. Refinement, however, strips these foods of most of their fiber and nutrients. Processing adds calories, subtracts nutrition, and contributes myriads of chemical additives. Strip seven pounds of sugar beets of their bulk, fiber, and nutrients, for instance, and you get one pound of pure sugar! Some 45 percent of the calories eaten are now "empty" calories, almost totally devoid of any significant nutritional value. No wonder many Americans are overfed and undernourished!

Cooked whole-grain cereals, rich in fiber, expand in your stomach, creating satiety, a feeling of fullness; and they save you money. On the other hand, presweetened cereals crumble and shrink to almost nothing, and they cost you, pound for pound of grain, eight to ten times more.

The least nutritious food with the most sugar is now the most widely advertised. Enormous resources of advertising go far toward the destruction of our more sensible eating habits. And don't forget that meat is the single largest source of fat in the U.S. diet, and its excess protein may contribute to kidney disease, gout, and osteoporosis. But even more serious is the heavy load of saturated fat that most animal protein foods carry, and the trans-fats found in crackers, cakes, pies, and crinkly bags, causing the liver to go into overdrive in making excessive cholesterol.

No wonder the surgeon general warned in *Nutrition and Health*: "For the two out of three adult Americans who do not smoke or drink excessively, one personal choice seems to influence long-term health prospects more than any other: what we eat."

Making the Change

Today, more than ever, we have become victims of our own lifestyle. The contribution of the medical care system to the health status of industrialized nations is marginal, since it can do little more than serve as a catchment net for those who have become victims of their own choices. The greatest health benefits are likely to accrue from efforts to improve the health habits of the American people instead of further medicalization of society.

Lifestyle Medicine Approach

So what would happen if people really simplified their diet, did something about their smoking, and started an exercise program? Since 1975 the Pritikin Longevity Center has had more than 75,000 people attend its residential one-to-four-week lifestyle-change program. More than 120 clinical reports sponsored by the Pritikin Research Foundation have been published in peer-reviewed journals demonstrating some of the advantages of a lifestyle medicine approach over the high-tech and pharmaceutical approaches, both in clinical outcomes and in cost-effectiveness.

Building on Pritikin's work, Dean Ornish, MD, then a young Harvard-trained cardiologist, published in 1990 the results of his randomized clinical trial with coronary patients in the Lancet Medical Journal. Employing a very simple, very low-fat, unrefined vegetarian diet coupled with exercise, stress management, and group support, he demonstrated with PET scans and angiography that the "majority of atherosclerotic lesions were indeed subject to regression regardless of the patient's age." These arterial lesions had actually begun to melt down.

Since then, his pioneering work has been duplicated, established, and extended in many clinical research centers around the world. For instance, Caldwell Esselstyn, Jr., MD, demonstrated at the Cleveland Clinic, in a twenty-year study, that diet alone (a simple, natural, vegetarian diet, very low in fat, sugar, and salt, yet high in fiber) could reverse coronary artery disease and dramatically reduce the incidence of subsequent coronary events! And Neal Barnard, MD, and many others, have demonstrated beyond the shadow of a doubt that a similar simple diet devoid of animal products was very effective in reversing T2 diabetes.

In addition, the clinical results of the Complete Health Improvement Program (CHIP) with more than 80,000 graduates of its four-to-twelve-week Intensive Therapeutic Lifestyle Change (ITLC) have demonstrated the efficacy of "lifestyle as medicine" in going beyond the mere symptomatic treatment of our common Western (chronic) diseases (www.CHIPhealth.com).

The Optimal Diet

An Optimal Diet, therefore, would emphasize the consumption of largely unrefined foods-as-grown. These foods, such as whole grains, legumes, vegetables and fresh fruit, are not only brimming with nutrients but are also high in fiber and volume, thus creating satiety without the caloric overloads. Therefore, they can be eaten freely without any concern for serving size. Of these foods: eat more, and you'll weigh less!

Such a natural whole-food diet—very low in fat and grease, animal protein, sugar and salt, yet high in fiber, antioxidants, and micronutrients and virtually free of cholesterol—is in stark contrast to the typically rich Western diet. Take a look at the chart on the next page (see Figure 3). Please note that the arrows pointing to "decrease" and "increase" for certain foods are dynamic in nature, which is indicated by the broken and progressive arrow design. This chart does not follow an ideologically prescribed dietary dogma. On the contrary, while it offers some optimal dietary reference points, it allows people to choose their level of implementation based on their motivation, clinical status, and readiness. Those in greatest need of clinical improvement do best by making the greatest dietary changes. For them, implementing a diet of simple whole foods (lots of fresh fruits and vegetables, whole grain products, and legumes, as well as some seeds and nuts) and devoid of any animal products offers the greatest clinical benefit and the potential to reverse disease.

Many people, as they begin to understand the cause-and-effect relationship between their dietary and lifestyle choices and the effects on their health and disease, give up the excesses of the "good life." Instead, they opt for the best life possible with its elegant simplicity. People, employees, executives, and administrators everywhere are making new commitments towards health, because while they realize that health may not be everything, they also recognize that without health, everything is nothing.

EAT FOR HEALTH!
Basic Guidelines for a Lifetime of Good Eating

EAT LESS

Fats and Oils

Strictly limit fatty meals, cooking and salad oils, sauces, dressings and shortening. Use margarine and nuts sparingly. Avoid frying (saute instead with a little water in nonstick pans. Especially avoid saturated and trans fats (cookies and crackers).

Sugars

Limit sugar, honey, molasses, syrups, pies, cakes, pastries, candy, cookies, soft drinks and sugar-rich desserts, such as pudding and ice cream. Save these foods for special occassions.

Cholesterol Foods

Progressively eliminate meat, sausages, egg yolks and liver. If used, limit dairy products to low-fat cheeses and nonfat milk products. If you eat fish and poultry, use them sparingly.

Salt

Use minimal salt during cooking. Banish the saltshaker. Strictly limit highly salted products, such as pickles, crackers, soy sauce, salted popcorn, nuts, chips, pretzels, and garlic salts.

Alcohol

Avoid alcohol in all forms, as well as caffeinated beverages, such as coffee, colas and black tea.

EAT MORE

Whole Grains

Freely use brown rice, millet, barley, corn, wheat, and rye. Also eat freely of whole-grain products, such as breads, pastas, shredded wheat and tortillas.

Tubers and Legumes

Freely use all kinds of potatoes and yams (without high-fat toppings). Enjoy peas, lentils, chickenpeas, and beans of every kind.

Fruits and Vegetables

Eat several fresh whole fruits every day. Limit fruits canned in syrup. Limit fiber-poor fruit juices. Eat a variety of vegetables daily. Enjoy fresh salads with low-calorie, low salt dressings.

Water

Drink eight glasses of water a day. Vary the routine with a twist of lemon and occasional herbal teas.

Hearty Breakfast
Enjoy hot multigrain cereals, fresh fruit, and whole-wheat toast. Jumpstart your day.

DIET COMPARISION

	U.S. Diet	*Optimal Diet*
Fats and Oils	80-120 g	under 45 g
Sugar	35 tsp	under 10 tsp
Cholesterol	400 mg	under 50 mg
Salt	10-15 g	under 5 g
Fiber	12 g	40 + g
Water Fluids	minimal	8 glasses

Figure 3 - (Adapted from the Optimal Diet by Hans Diehl)

THE POWER OF CHOICE

By Co-Editors Joyce & Linda

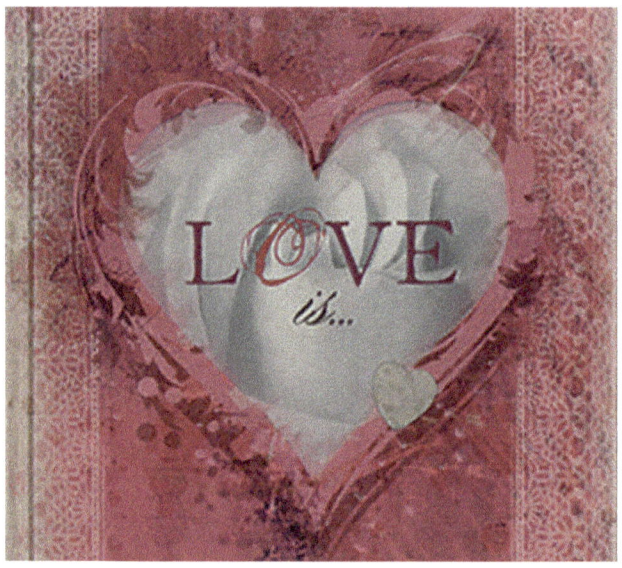

The Power of Choice begins with Love! And it's this genuine love that gives meaning to our lives, which then radiates and transforms our world. It's a mysterious and magical joy that brightens our lives and becomes the greatest treasure of all. But it's only known to those who truly love.

Our passion and mission is to create opportunities that will transform people's lives through evidence-based nutrition and intelligent self-care, thus facilitating total health and vibrant living!

Many people today are concerned about their health. Yet many have already been afflicted by the growing epidemic of our modern killer diseases, for which high tech medicine can only offer symptomatic relief with rarely arresting or reversing and curing these chronic diseases. The reason is because these diseases are not related to some pathogen or bug that could be eliminated with some antibiotic medication. These diseases are related to our culturally promoted lifestyle and our lifestyle habits—prominently among them, a rich diet, smoking, and sedentary living.

Some 100 years ago, these chronic diseases were rare. Sir William Osler, MD, professor of medicine at Johns Hopkins University in Baltimore wrote in his 1928 published text book: "When it comes to heart attacks, you can expect one heart attack per year in an average hospital in an average-sized American town." Today, the number of heart attacks in the US is 3,000 per day with cardiovascular disease being responsible for every third death.

Similarly, the most common form of diabetes has increased by over 400 percent over the last thirty years. This is now making every second American adult either a diabetic or one with pre-diabetes at risk for becoming a full-blown diabetic. At the same time, obesity since 1985 has increased from under 10 percent in the American adult population to 35 percent currently.

These chronic disease trends have been associated with a major shift in the food supply. Our diet and culture have changed. We have gone from eating at home to eating out. We have gone from slow foods to fast foods. Oats have turned into Oreos, potatoes into Pringles, corn into Doritos, beans into burgers, and water has turned in soda and Monster drinks.

The purpose for putting this book together is to share stories of how individuals' lives have been transformed from poor health and disease to living healthy, vibrant lives simply by making better dietary choices and by placing a higher priority on their health. We hope these stories will uplift our readers and awaken hope to make dietary changes consistent with the optimum functioning of our bodies and to prevent, arrest, and facilitate the reversal of many of these common killer diseases. We can do more for ourselves in fighting these lifestyle-related diseases than any doctor, pill, or hospital.

Our goal is to inspire a large awakening towards a higher level of health consciousness that will empower the readers to make changes to live a more balanced, healthy, and meaningful life. We believe it's time for us to "fight the war against these largely culturally promoted and oftentimes self-chosen diseases."

Our collective health stories have taken us both along the high road and the low road. We have experienced major health issues. We had to deal with traumatic family losses and seemingly insurmountable stress. We had to deal with fearful illnesses in our children. But we got through those tunnels of turmoil. We did not give up. Instead, we faced those challenges and turned our scars into stars. Our individual journeys taught us that we can accomplish whatever we set our minds to do. In the process, we began to recognize that health was the foundation in rebuilding our lives and the lives of our children and loved ones. And it's our heartfelt desire to share this newfound level of health and wholeness with our readers.

We believe that we have been designed to live our lives in balance, where plant-based whole foods play a major role in contributing to our health and healing instead of relying primarily on medication with all of their side effects, high costs, and their lack of affecting a cure for most of these modern killer diseases.

Could it be that many of us have fallen short of what our Creator-God had intended for us in living our lives closer to natural foods? Many thoughtful leading voices are now talking about our lifestyle choices, our fast-paced living, and our environment that all have taken their toll on our health as well as on Planet Earth, which many now consider in "survival mode." We are all at difference stages of our health journey. As we transition to living a more balanced, healthy life, it is our desire to provide guidance to help you choose to live a more health-filled you.

It's NOW time for us to take our health back and to combine our energies in fighting the war against this chronic disease epidemic. As co-editors, we have put this book together to inspire and help you to discover your own personal health journey. It is our hearts' desire to partner with you, our reader, to have you join us in our passion and mission for changing lives by helping others to make lifestyle and habit changes that will have positive lasting results for you and your loved ones.

We invite you to share in this amazing journey with us and choose to live a healthy, vibrant life. After all, most health is not so much a matter of chance, as it is more commonly a matter of choice.

Love is misunderstood to be an emotion. Actually it is a state of awareness, a way of being in the world, a way of seeing oneself and others.

Dr. David R. Hawkins

BATTLEFIELD OF THE MIND

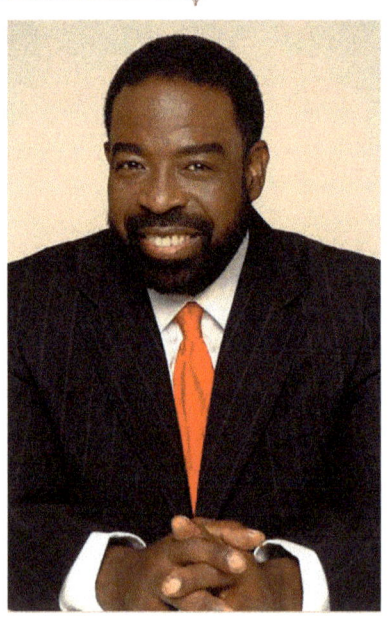

Les Brown

In the wake of massive success and many tremendous accomplishments I have experienced in nearly thirty-five years of professional speaking, one of the hardest things for me to believe was that I could do it. I've had to continuously convince myself that not only do I deserve what I have, but what I have achieved is only a tip of the iceberg of what is possible for me. As far back as I can remember, I have had to overcome the stigma of low expectations with an inner knowing that I was more than someone's opinion of me. I have been able to outlive all the negative labels that society has tried to pin on me. My biggest challenge has been to overcome the negative inner conversation I speak to myself, which I call "The Battlefield of the Mind," and the war waged is for my destiny.

After being diagnosed with cancer over a decade ago, my goal has been to maintain a healthy body and live my life cancer-free. I have been blessed because many people die from the prognosis of the disease rather than the disease itself. I realize that there are certain things I need to do to reach that goal, such as not eating sugar. As much as I may like sweets, I know that cancer feeds off sugar. I'm still here because I chose to fight rather than give up and accept what doctors have told me. My adopted mother had breast cancer and was a survivor for over twenty years, so I know the importance of keeping a healthy regimen. I also know that I need a good physical exercise program.

Fortunately, I realize at this stage in my life that I can no longer delude myself by saying that I am too busy or don't have enough time to develop a regular exercise regimen, when one of my main goals is to take better care of myself. I have always said, "Nothing tastes as good as health feels."

After years of seeking information and trying to learn as much as I can about health, I know that there is no magical formula to getting and maintaining good health. However contrary to the knowledge I have gained, it is still a battle for me to do what I know to do. Paul, in my favorite book said, "The good that I should do, I don't do, and the very thing I hate, that I do." I can truly relate to his struggle, because too often it is my struggle as well. However, in my case, I realize that I can no longer try to reach my desired level of health while keeping such a fast-paced lifestyle.

There is a sense of inner power that we get when we cannot hear from anyone else but God. I need to be silent so that I can become centered and reconnect with my source of true power. That's how to win "The Battlefield of the Mind."

This has been Mrs. Mamie Brown's baby boy, Leslie Calvin Brown. That's my story, and I'm sticking to it!

Les Brown, Author

Motivational Speaker
www.lesbrown.com
Facebook.com/brown.les

Les Brown has authorized the co-editors of *Loving Healthy Living* to use all or part of the excerpt from a book project by Valorie N. Parker, *Unveiling Secrets from the Heart*.

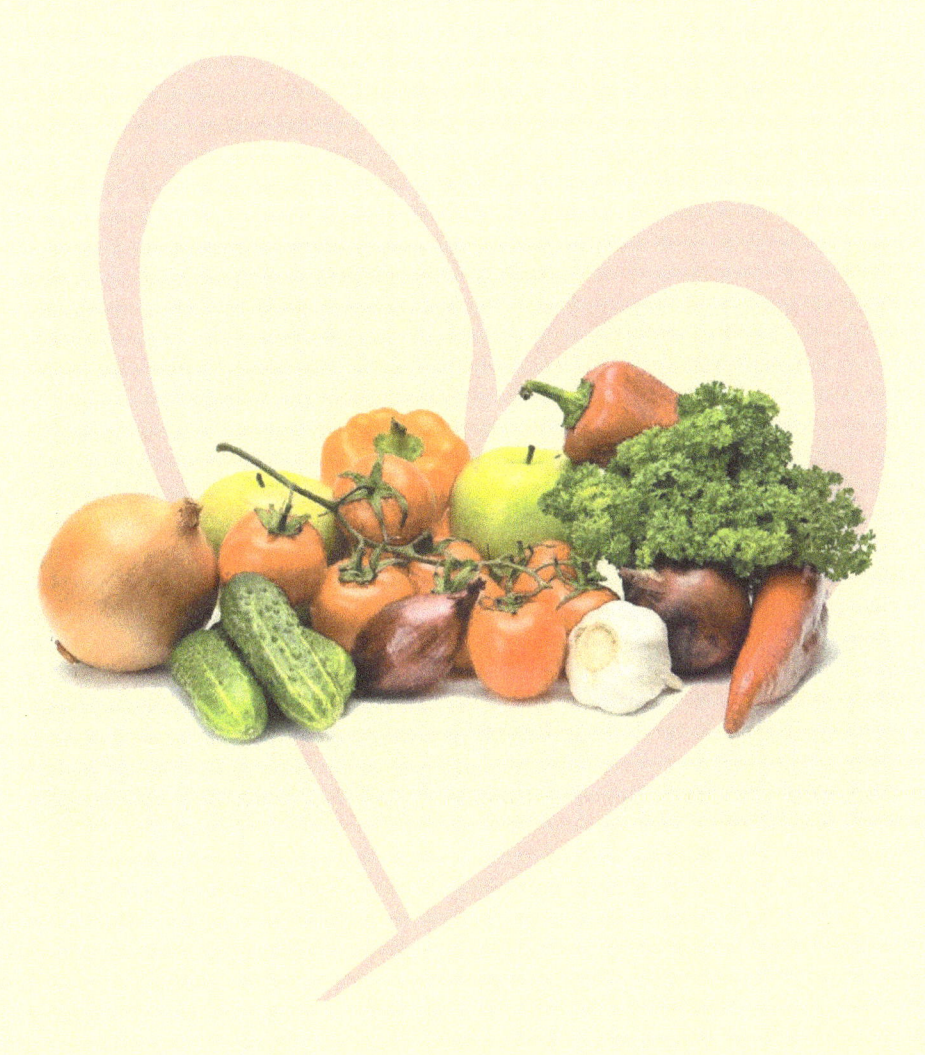

A RETURN TO LOVE

Marianne Williamson

Our deepest fear is not that we are inadequate.
Our deepest fear is that we are powerful beyond measure.
It is our light, not our darkness, that most frightens us.
We ask ourselves, who am I to be brilliant, gorgeous,
talented and fabulous?
Actually, who are you not to be?
You are a child of God
Your playing small doesn't serve the world.
There is nothing enlightened about shrinking so that
other people won't feel insecure around you.
We were born to manifest the glory of
God that is within us.
It's not just in some of us; it's in everyone.
And as we let our own light shine, we unconsciously
give other people permission to do the same.
As we are liberated from our own fears, our presence
automatically liberates others.

LOVE IS BEAUTIFUL

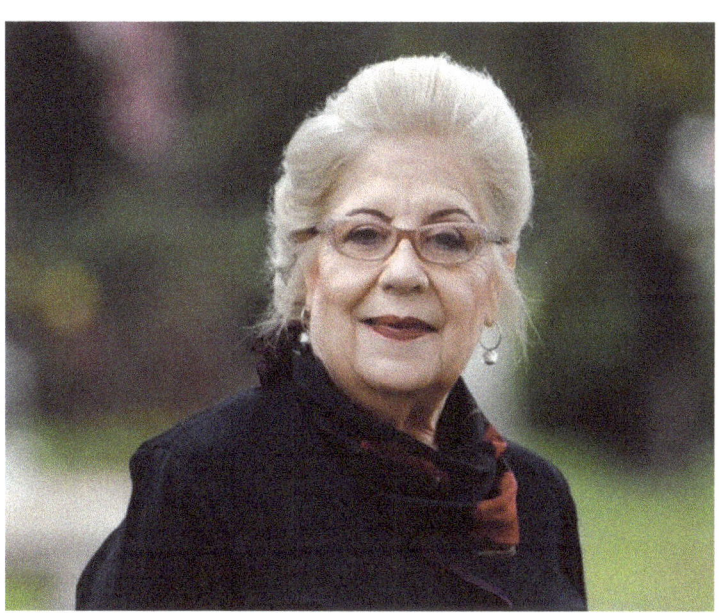

Joyce Hack

Born in Manitoba, Canada, I grew up on a farm with five sisters. My twin sister and I were the oldest. Farm life was difficult, and to survive you had to work hard. At age seven, I was already babysitting my younger siblings and learning how to prepare meals. At age eight, I was already making breads, cookies, and cakes.

Cooking at such an early age and making a difference in my family's life was the beginning of my journey to care for and to make a difference in the lives of others. I remember buying little gifts of love for my sisters and my parents. Recognizing that my mother never had a bedspread—

she used homemade quilts—I used my first paycheck to purchase my mom her first bedspread. And she never forgot it. When she passed in her ninety-eighth year, we found that bedspread I had given her some seventy years ago in her trunk where she kept some of her precious things.

As time passed, my passion became healthy, nutritious cooking. My first instructor was my precious mother. She was an excellent cook. Many of her dishes were made from scratch and without any recipes. Our large garden yielded an abundance of produce that we canned and froze and turned into jams, marmalade, and jellies. At the same time, we took advantage of the fruits that grew wild around our farm. There were Saskatoon berries, cranberries, strawberries, gooseberries and the best rhubarb. These fruits growing in God's garden always seemed to be the best. I especially remember a recipe my mother and I created using wild cranberries in making ketchup that was out of this world and became a favorite topping for meats, stews, and just about every food.

Life on the farm was not easy: milking cows, cleaning manure from the barn, feeding the animals, doing chores. It became obvious to me that I needed to create a different future for myself. And so, at the age of seventeen, I left home and moved to Winnipeg, the largest city in Manitoba. I got my first job at the Marlborough Hotel as a salad and sandwich dietary aide. As several of the chefs saw my passion for food preparation, they began to mentor me. Although working at the hotel full time, I did my grade twelve at night school. And upon completion of my senior matriculation and my experience at the Marlborough Hotel, I decided to become a chef.

I did my culinary training at the Red River Community College, followed by a one-year apprenticeship at the Winnipeg Health Science Center. It was here that the director of nutritional services gave me the opportunity to not only train cooks and bakers but to also become a certified food service manager. As a very thoughtful and inspiring mentor, she took me aside one day and encouraged and challenged me: "How about getting trained as a registered dietitian?" It was a recommendation that stayed with me.

Several years later, I married my husband who had a nursing degree. As a very adventurous young couple, and after doing our homework, we decided to move to California. Our oldest daughter was then three years old, and I was pregnant with our second daughter.

That challenge given to me years ago now came into focus. I was going to become a registered dietitian. I was going to enroll in the nutrition program at Loma Linda University, a well-respected health-centered institution with a large teaching hospital. The university had an excellent nutrition program with cutting-edge researchers. I was going to do it!

But then, shortly after starting my degree program, my husband was killed in a motorcycle accident that changed everything. In an instant, I became a single mother with two small children. I thought of quitting school and moving back to the safety of Canada. After all, it is very difficult to fully understand the "whys of any of these tragedies." Yet somehow the loving heart seems to keep growing not just in spite of but often because of these painful experiences, marshaling the development of often unknown resources, such as tolerance, courage, and goal-orientation.

But after a brief mourning period, I knew that I couldn't do that. I just couldn't give up on my dreams of higher education, healthcare, and helping others. The road before me was clear. It would be a rough ride, because not only did I have to provide for my little family—financially, emotionally, physically, and spiritually—but I also had to find ways to pursue my professional dreams. With flexible working hours in the food service area of a nursing home, plus some excellent mentorship and guidance from friends and professors, and with many long hours and late nights, I felt overjoyed when, five years later, I graduated as a registered dietitian. It was a never to be forgotten moment of triumph and a lesson for my young daughters. Never give up. Believe in yourself and in miracles.

I am now offering thirty-five years of professional experience in clinical nutrition and management. As an effective leader committed to positive outcomes in all aspects of life, I inspire others by showing thoughtfulness and kindness. That's why some have called me the secret ingredient in a recipe of inspiration. As such, my greatest joy is to encourage people to improve their lifestyle and health, and to inspire them to live more balanced and meaningful lives.

As I am now embarking on this new journey as a health coach certified by the Health Coach Institute, I feel excited that in the last chapter of my life, I can offer my unique talents and gifts to changing not only the health of people but also their consciousness of a planet in survival mode. Based on cutting-edge psychology, brain science, and personal growth, our curriculum as health coaches is designed to effectively help people to improve their lives and to facilitate total health.

My motto is "Love with an uninhibited soul and make a triumph of every aspect of your life." I am looking forward to working with you on your journey of triumphs. Let me help you, as I will show you how to believe in miracles and in yourself.

> Nothing of great value in life comes
> easily. The things of
> highest value come hard.
> The gold that has the greatest value
> lies deepest in the earth,
> as do diamonds.

Norman Vincent Peale

Joyce Hack, RDN

Certified Health Coach
Redlands, California
www.feelingfabulousoverfifty.com
Joyinred@verizon.net
www.5linx.net/jhack (click on opportunity)

QUINOA SALAD

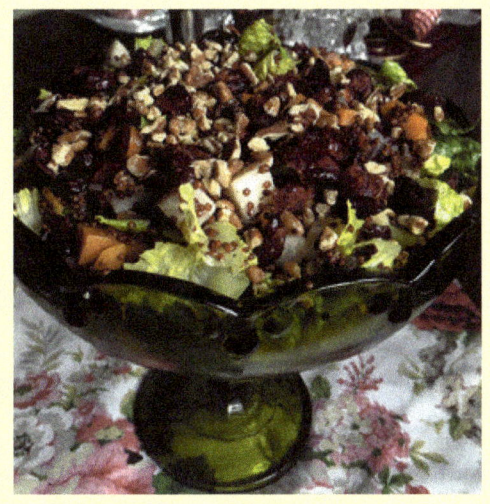

Calories	335
Protein	5g
CHO	41g
Fat	18g
Sugar	17g
Sodium	300mg
Fiber	5g
Chol	0mg

Per serving, serves 6

INGREDIENTS

Apple Cider Vinaigrette

- 1 cup apple juice
- 1 tablespoon shallot, finely diced
- 1 tablespoon fresh thyme leaves
- 1 tablespoon dijon-style mustard
- ¼ cup apple cider vinegar
- ¼ cup olive oil
- ¼ cup Granny Smith apple, finely diced
- ¼ teaspoon freshly ground black pepper

Salad

- 1 cup quinoa
- salt, finely ground
- 1 medium carrot, cut into ¼-inch cubes
- ½ medium yellow onion, finely chopped
- ½ cup jicama, cut into ¼-inch cubes
- ½ teaspoon finely chopped fresh rosemary
- ¼ teaspoon dried sage
- 2 cups romaine lettuce, chopped medium pieces
- ½ cup toasted pecans, chopped
- ½ cup dried cranberries, roughly chopped

DIRECTIONS

For the vinaigrette: Pour the apple juice into a small saucepan. Add the shallot and thyme, place over medium-high heat, bring to a boil, and boil until juice reduced in volume by two-thirds, about 10 minutes. Pour into a bowl and set aside to cool to room temperature. Whisk in the mustard, followed by the vinegar, then slowly whisk in the oil until emulsified. Stir in the apple and pepper.

For the salad: Preheat the oven to 350°F. Put the quinoa on a baking sheet, place in the oven, and toast, stirring a couple of times, for 10 minutes, or until fragrant and golden in color.

Meanwhile, fill a large bowl with ice and water to make an ice-water bath. Fill a large saucepan with water and bring to a boil over high heat. Salt the water, then add the carrot and onion and cook for 2 to 3 minutes, until crisp-tender. Remove the vegetables with a slotted spoon and briefly submerge them in the ice-water bath to stop the cooking. Remove from the ice-water bath to a plate and pat dry with paper towels.

Return the water to a boil, add the quinoa, and cook for about 10 minutes, until the quinoa just starts to open into a tiny curl. Strain the quinoa through a fine-mesh sieve and briefly rinse under cold water. Drain well. Transfer to a serving bowl, add the blanched vegetable, the jicama, rosemary, and sage, and toss with ¼ cup of the dressing (reserve the rest for another salad). Add the romaine and toss to coat well in the dressing. Add the pecans and cranberries, taste, and add more salt and pepper if needed. Spoon into bowls and serve.

Chef's Note: Salad is high in nutrients and inexpensive. It's a great source of fiber, it's gluten-free, and it's a complete protein. Since this 7,000-year-old grain is so bland, it takes on the flavor of whatever it's cooked with. Don't be afraid to play around. I prefer to cook it in vegetable stock. It is also a nice oatmeal substitute if you toast it first and then cook it with cinnamon and apples.

ROASTED EGGPLANT WITH KALE, FRESH MOZZARELLA, & PINE NUTS

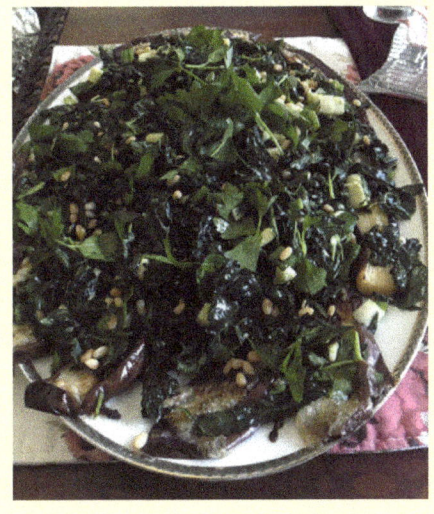

Calories	289
Protein	17g
CHO	25g
Fat	7g
Sugar	9g
Sodium	350mg
Fiber	13g
Chol	6mg

Per serving, serves 6

INGREDIENTS

- 6 baby eggplants (about 6 inches long)
- pinch salt
- ½ bunch Tuscan kale
- 1 tablespoon olive oil
- 2 cloves garlic, grated
- 2 ounces fresh mozzarella cheese, cut into small cubes
- ½ cup currants
- ½ cup fresh basil, chopped
- ¼ cup flat-leaf parsley leaves, chopped
- ½ cup green onions, sliced
- 2 teaspoons balsamic cream*
- pinch black pepper, freshly cracked
- 4 tablespoons pine nuts, toasted

DIRECTIONS

Preheat the oven to 425°F. Slice the eggplant in half lengthwise and place cut side up on a baking sheet. Spritz with cooking spray, sprinkle with salt, and roast for 20 minutes, or until lightly browned.

Meanwhile, remove the stems from the kale, stack the leaves, and thinly slice them. Sprinkle the leaves with ¼ teaspoon salt and rub it in with your hands. Let sit for 10 minutes so the leaves can start to soften.

In a small bowl, combine the oil and garlic. Add garlic oil to the kale and mix well to coat the leaves. Fold in the cheese, currants, basil, parsley, and chives. Place the eggplant on a plate and drizzle with balsamic cream and a little salt and pepper. Top with the kale salad, sprinkle on the pine nuts, and serve.

Chef's Note: Serve it with a bowl of soup, and lunch is ready to go! Tuscan kale is also known as "black kale" and "Lacinato kale." *Balsamic cream is a prepared item that comes in a jar, available for purchase at Trader Joes or online health food retailers.

HEALTHY CHOICES
HEALTHY LIFE

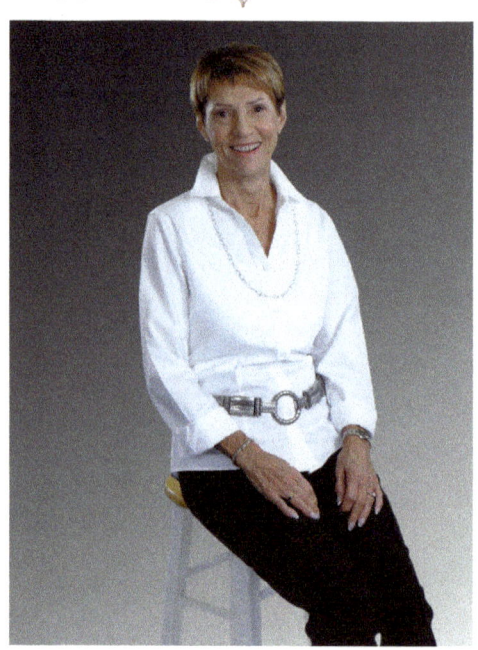

Linda McLeod

Health and good nutrition were part of my life from an early age. I was very fortunate to grow up in Saskatoon, Saskatchewan, where my father would spend his summers growing a fabulous garden that provided excellent produce for our family all year round. My upbringing and heritage taught me a great deal about living healthy. When as a child I became very ill with hepatitis, our home was quarantined, physicians visited me every day, and once diagnosed, the recovery was painstakingly slow. Although I missed an entire year of school, I gradually recovered, largely because my parents fed me natural, healthy, whole foods, which helped in my recovery and in my staying healthy.

When I left home, I found it more difficult to maintain those choices because of a very busy work life. And because foods-as-grown were often harder to find (the organic food industry had not yet emerged), I did not always make the best food choices. My work schedule was very hectic as I traveled around British Columbia and throughout Canada for IBM. And, as a result, I had to face another major health crisis. Hospitalized for several months, I made a big decision. I would live as healthily as possible. I was going to do what I had learned. I adapted a plant-strong healthy diet. I did fasting and cleansing regularly to not only recover my health but also to better manage my weight. And I made a commitment that I would not return to my many yo-yo diets. But that was often easier said than done …

Regrettably, after ten years of marriage, I found myself raising three small children on my own. Even so, I was committed to raising these children in the best way I could. Happily, this worked out (for the most part), in that my children are my best friends today. But then I had to face another challenge: during my thirteen years as a single parent, I found myself in a situation with my oldest son who was having a very difficult time. I wanted to find a solution for him, so I took him to several specialists, all to no avail. Nothing was working. At last, when he was in grade ten—now in his second school—he was diagnosed with Attention Deficit Hyperactivity Disorder (ADHD). Discounting the benefits of a change in diet, the physicians instead recommended Ritalin. My response, however, was an emphatic *no*. Instead of Ritalin, I would first try a dietary makeover. And I did: I removed all dairy and sugar from his regular diet. What an unbelievable difference that made! I finally had a son who was calm. I had a son who loved school. I now had a son who achieved in sports and finally loving his life. Today, he is an amazing artist and digital animator. Plus, I might add, he is a wonderful cook.

But then I had to face another major health challenge in my own life, possibly the result of all the stress I had been through. Diagnosed with pneumonia, but without proper treatment by several physicians over the next two years, this pneumonia turned into a very serious lung disease. With little hope for recovery, the best my pulmonary specialist could do was recommend antibiotics for the rest of my life. Not finding this an acceptable choice or option, I remembered the good food choices my parents taught me. I decided to go back to the basics of what I practiced in the past plus what I learned from doctors who offered alternative medicine. As a result, I continued down this path rather than follow the recommendations of my more traditional physicians. Admittedly, it was not easy. It was an uphill battle for a time. But with persistence and determination to recover my health once more, I went back to a simpler, natural whole food program augmented with some supplements provided by my alternative medical support team.

It's been quite a journey. It has taught me many lessons about health, about life, and about making the best choices in difficult health situations. Today, I live my life in a more balanced form. My food pattern is centered in natural, organic, food-as-grown that is simply prepared. I love to cook. And I love to take care of others. And I am happy to say that my lung condition is completely healed.

In the process, health has become my passion. Nothing gives me more joy than to pass on some of the knowledge I have acquired over the years and to see the transformation in women's lives. Too long, many of us have underestimated the power of the body's ability to heal itself, provided we treat it right.

I am truly excited for the privilege of being able to focus on women's health and to help women transform their lives through healthy habits and good nutrition. With the challenges I have met successfully in my own life, and with the validation I have received as a certified health & wellness coach, I have found my niche in empowering women to transform their lives through mind and body wellness and through the establishment of better health habits. I am here to help them to identify the symptoms, to diagnose the cause, and to provide solutions and then teach and motivate them to recover their health, to feel fabulous and energized and to feel once more in charge of their lives and health and ready to live more.

I provide the right system, the support, and the accountability that will make a difference in your life, and you can experience the same results that others have already experienced. If what you are doing is no longer working and you are looking for something greater to get where you want to go, then contact me. In the meanwhile, however, my friend and colleague Joyce and I hope that this amazing book of stories will warm your heart and that the wonderful recipes from all contributors will help facilitate a healthier you.

> Habits are like financial capital—forming one today is an investment that will automatically give out returns for years to come.

Shawn Anchor

Linda McLeod

Certified Health & Lifestyle Coach
Coquitlam, British Columbia
www.healthhabits4life.com
linda@healthhabits4life.com

GREEN BEANS & RED PEPPER SIDE DISH

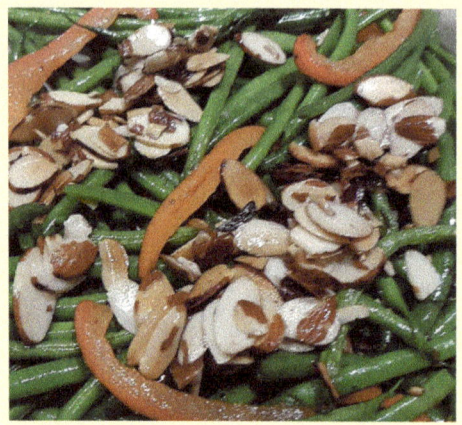

Calories	335
Protein	5g
CHO	41g
Fat	18g
Sugar	17g
Sodium	378mg
Fiber	5g
Chol	0mg

Per serving

Serves 4

INGREDIENTS

- 3 cups fresh green beans
- 1 medium size red pepper, deseeded and sliced thin to match the size of the beans (use orange or yellow if you prefer)
- 2 green onions, sliced into rounds
- 2 large garlic cloves cut into small pieces
- ¼ cup of sliced roasted almonds
- pinch of Himalayan salt
- pinch of ground black pepper
- ⅓ tablespoon olive or avocado oil

DIRECTIONS

In a pan over medium heat, bring water to boiling. Add beans to boiling water, then cook 3 minutes until bright green and slightly softened. If you like crunchy green beans, monitor cooking time and check your green beans while cooking.

Slice red pepper into long narrow pieces to match the size of the beans.

Place oil in pan and lightly fry green onions and garlic. Place partially cooked beans and red peppers in with onion mixture. Cook for 2–3 minutes and season with salt and black pepper to taste.

Just before serving, sprinkle sliced almonds over top.

WILD RICE AND STUFFED ACORN SQUASH

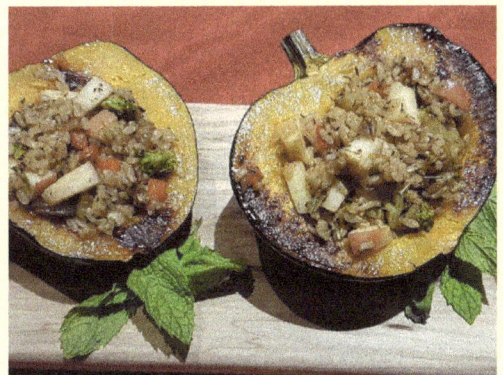

Calories	210
Protein	3g
CHO	5g
Fat	6g
Sugar	6g
Sodium	35mg
Fiber	6g
Chol	0mg

Makes 4 servings

Per serving

INGREDIENTS

- ¼ cup wild rice, rinsed
- 2 small acorn squash, halved and cored
- 1 tablespoon plus 2 teaspoons olive or avocado oil
- ½ cup finely chopped onion
- 2 garlic cloves, finely chopped
- 2 celery stalks, diced
- 1 large red apple, unpeeled and diced
- 1 tablespoon fresh thyme

DIRECTIONS

In a glass metal bowl, cover wild rice with 1 cup boiling water. Let sit covered for 1 hour, until kernels pop and then drain water.

Preheat oven to 400°F.

Brush inside of each squash half with ½ teaspoon olive or avocado oil.

Place squash flat side down on a parchment-lined baking sheet. Bake 30 minutes or until squash is tender.

Five minutes before squash is finished cooking, prepare stuffing. In nonstick skillet, sauté onion, garlic, and celery in remaining oil over medium-high heat for about 3 minutes. Add apple; cook 2 minutes. Add rice and thyme, mix well.

Remove squash from oven and stuff with wild rice blend. Serve warm.

THE YUM STORY

How Living Deliciously Can Become a Way of Life[1]

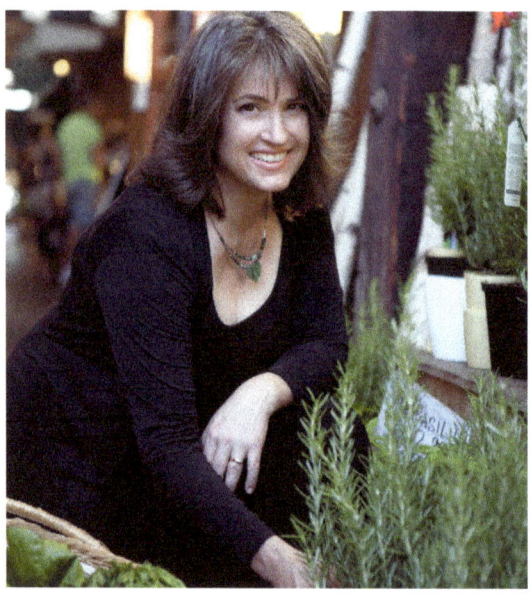

Theresa Nicasso

In 1995, I married my long-time, beloved friend, Eric Mazzi. Together, we were moving along in life with our dog and three cats, just like so many others. Then something unexpected happened that profoundly changed the trajectory of my life: I got pregnant! It wasn't that the

---

[1] (Excerpt from award-winning *YUM: Plant-based Recipes for a Gluten-free Diet*, by Theresa Nicassio PhD, Sept 2015)

pregnancy was unexpected—it had been planned for and hoped for, and was a wonderful blessing. What was unexpected were the consequences of my pregnancy: physical debilitation and a cascade of health problems that lasted for more than a decade after our daughter Alex's birth in 1997.

What the heck! I say this jokingly now, but—believe me—it was no joke. In fact, it was downright terrifying at times. My immune and respiratory systems began to fail, neurological problems and chronic pain reduced my mobility and general functioning, and my life became a battle against perpetual infection, inflammation, fatigue, weight gain, and an endless list of food and environmental sensitivities. Medical appointments and visits to the hospital became a major focus of my existence, but all the while, I was still trying to be a good mom and contributing member of society in my professional capacity.

I knew this was not how I wanted to spend the rest of my life, but no matter how hard I tried, my condition only worsened. If it hadn't been for my meditation practice, my rebellious spirit of hope, my loving partner, our beautiful children, and the gift of meaningful work, I don't know how I could have survived and functioned as well as I did. My belief in the body's natural tendency and desire to heal itself was activated during this time and was a great blessing. A fire in my gut propelled me to fight against my condition; it felt like a force more powerful than I could have mustered alone, and I embraced it. I chose to fight for a cause. I chose to say "yes" to life in all its forms and advocate for it, starting with the little world I was in—first my body, then my family, and then beyond.

Somehow I was given the courage and tenacity to search for a way to transform myself and to emerge from this suffering. You name the treatment (even unmentionable ones I would never wish on anyone), I probably tried it. Most treatments, whether conventional or alternative, resulted in minimal or no benefit at best, and not-so-attractive side effects at worst. I'd enthusiastically complied with countless caring and competent professionals' advice, yet my health didn't improve and the chronic conditions and negative effects of some of my medications continued to worsen. I knew that something needed to change, but what? It was just one big mystery. I had met my Baba Yaga in a big way!

At a certain point, I realized that it was I who had to be the agent of change. The well-intentioned medical professionals at the time were unable to help, so I had to take responsibility for learning about my body in a whole new way. While I didn't know where to start, my lifelong love of science became my best ally. It was time to pull out all the stops and become my own case study. I took every conventional and alternative course about health and healing that I could, and became immersed in a journey of discovery that has changed my world forever.

While in the midst of all this research and experimentation, I reconnected with my former colleague and friend from the University of British Columbia, Dr. Hal Gunn. Hal and I had shared a passion for honoring the mind-body-spirit connection and a belief in the body's innate capacity to heal itself. He had followed his dream as a physician by co-founding an innovative holistic and integrative cancer treatment centre in Vancouver, Inspire Health, with Dr. Roger Rodgers in 1997. During our visit, Hal gave me Inspire Health's comprehensive, research-based information package that contained resources to empower their patients living with cancer. One of the things that stood out most for me, as I later perused the centre's materials, was the section about foods that help to fight cancer. This excited me and launched my curiosity about how food could be used as medicine—and how healthy organic food, from naturally enriched soil, as fresh as possible (ideally grown at or near your own home) can be even better medicine.

Another great discovery I made was the work of Functional Medicine pioneers who spoke about how the wrong food for an individual can result in an inner world of toxicity. I learned more about the role of environmental and food allergies and cross-allergens, as well as how food sensitivities contribute to inflammation. Reading and employing Dr. Natasha Turner's book, *The Hormone Diet*, was a pivotal point in my journey. Her book opened my eyes to the barrage of toxins I had been exposed to—in food, air and water—and how hard my body had been working to cope with these assaults. Natasha's book also introduced me to a simple elimination program to identify food sensitivities. Through this process, I discovered that when I completely eliminated gluten from my diet, the migraine headaches (from which I'd suffered all my life) disappeared. And the pain that filled every part of my body also lessened—all in less than a month! Holy cow—was that really possible? After all the treatments I had tried, this was the first clear improvement I experienced. It did not resolve all of my symptoms by any stretch, but it made a significant dent.

Okay, I was hooked.

Also in 2010, Alex—then twelve years old—saw Alicia Silverstone (actor and author of *The Kind Diet*) on The Oprah Winfrey Show talking about how farm animals are treated. After watching that program, Alex became a vegan in less than a week. Boom! How we ate as a family took another dramatic turn overnight.

Then there was the 2011 release of Dr. William Davis's *Wheat Belly*, a book that rocked the world. In it, Davis blew the whistle on wheat and demonstrated the connection between wheat and heart disease, diabetes, celiac disease, weight gain, the aging process, and a host of neurological problems. Both Dr. David Perlmutter, in his book *Grain Brain*, and Dr. Alessio Fasano, in his book *Gluten Freedom*, have subsequently brought more research findings about gluten and its potential health implications to light. For the first time since Drs. Colin and Thomas Campbell's 2005 book, *The China Study*, which linked diet with chronic illness and mortality, the public was whacked in the gut in a way that could no longer be ignored.

In an effort to care for the needs of all our family members, Alex and I started trying a huge range of plant-based, gluten-free and sugar-free foods in 2010. But we had a problem: most of them tasted terrible to us. So we started to read every recipe book we could get our hands on, as well as countless recipes from the internet, with only a few successes. We were able to find some products and recipes that were either vegan or gluten-free that we liked, but rarely any that were both. Those we did try were often filled with refined sugar, margarine, and other ingredients that we prefer to avoid. After a year of major frustration, we realized that we had to create our own recipes if we wanted to enjoy food that met our standards for health and taste.

Ever so slowly, we were able to come up with delicious meals that reflected the high quality flavor, texture, and appearance that we sought—and were also easy and quick to make, given our busy lives.

It was amazing. When Alex and I decided to sink our teeth (so to speak) into taking on this challenge, it was impossible to stop us. Despite many culinary failures along the way, we were super excited when we had finally developed enough recipes to be able to once again invite friends over for meals—unapologetically. Yeah!

Then in 2013, Alex and I decided to go to the Living Light International Culinary Institute in California to learn even more. That year, we became Associate Raw Food Chefs and Instructors. I went back in 2014 to complete the Gourmet Raw Food Chef program, and then later that same year, Alex and I returned for the Advanced Raw Food Nutrition Educator Certification program.

We've now become a resource for others, sharing our recipes with friends who have similar dietary challenges. We are not alone; it was mind-blowing to learn how many folks live with food limitations!

Most people are tired of hearing about what they "need to," "ought to," "have to," or "should" be eating—or what they should be feeding their kids—because of health problems. I have found that such pressure not only results in very little sustainable behaviour change, but all too often also results in undue stress and guilt that serves no one. I want you to be able to shed any despair, frustration, or self-blame so that you are less likely to give up if you don't feel able to resist eating food that you know may be harmful to your body.

When grace and love are invited in, shame and hopelessness fade. When this happens, like a seed inspired to sprout and thrive, you'll find yourself better able to make life-enhancing choices, almost effortlessly.

As a psychologist, I have absolutely no interest or desire in colluding with potentially harmful ways of thinking.

My passion runs deep, both personally and as a professional who has practiced psychotherapy for almost thirty years. So, while writing a cookbook is the last thing I ever imagined I might be doing, it is clearly what I have been called to do. And while an unlikely vehicle for my life path, this philosophically grounded project indisputably resonates with my heartfelt commitment to do what I can to help others suffer less.

This is a world I know extremely well. It was the inspirational guiding force that gave me the tenacity to develop this extensive collection of recipes. For years, I saw my beloved dad struggling with diabetes, heart disease, kidney failure, and the associated circulation issues and neuropathy. Witnessing his struggles around food, which only worsened in his last years of life, was heart-wrenching. I'll never forget how he couldn't stop himself from eating the delicious cake at his granddaughter's birthday party, just days before the first of four amputation surgeries on both his legs. He died one year later, after living with unbearable pain every moment of that year. I want to help prevent you and countless others from having to live through such agony, and at the same time make it possible for everyone to enjoy the pleasure of sharing celebrations with loved ones—including being able to savour every bite of delectable cake at your granddaughter's birthday, or graduation, or wedding. With the alarming increase in the rates of obesity and diabetes (especially for our youth), my longing to help turn the boat around couldn't be stronger. The great news is that delicious food doesn't have to wreak havoc on our bodies—it's time to shed that outmoded belief.

Go ahead, call me crazy, because I am—crazy about life, crazy about love, and now, more than ever, crazy about delicious and non-toxic food that nourishes instead of harms my body and the planet. It hasn't been easy, but it fills my heart with indescribable joy to be able to transform my struggle and frustration into an opportunity to create something worthwhile for others, something that might help bring to your life, and the lives of others, a little more ease.

Theresa Nicassio, PhD, Psychologist

Registered Psychologist #1451
Award-Winning Bestselling Author
Host of The Dr. Theresa Nicassio Show
Gourmet Raw Food Chef & Advanced Raw Food Nutrition Educator
TheresaNicassio.com

CREAMY CARROT & GINGER SOUP

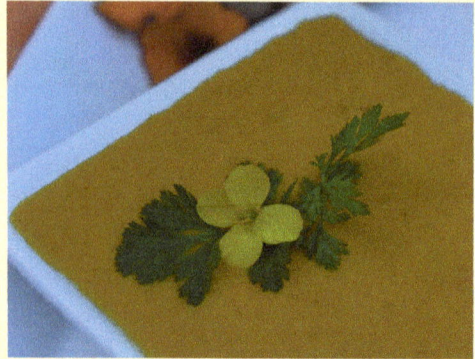

Calories	346
Protein	5g
CHO	41g
Fat	18g
Sugar	17g
Sodium	378mg
Fiber	5g
Chol	0mg

Makes 5 servings

It was a longstanding dream of mine to make a soup like this. Once I managed it, it was even more incredible than I had hoped! In devising this recipe, I was committed to making it super-simple, so when I had the brainstorm to roast roughly chopped vegetables, I got really excited. I also love that I found a way to use cilantro stems, which otherwise end up in the compost.

This soup is sure to be a crowd-pleaser, filled with ingredients that most people have on hand and that most people, even those with allergies and auto-immune conditions, are able to eat. The only problem is that it doesn't last long: If you want to have leftovers or will be serving guests, you might consider doubling or tripling the recipe. If you do so, you'll need to blend it in batches.

INGREDIENTS

- 2 cups carrots, roughly chopped
- 1 small or medium yellow onion, roughly chopped
- 2 celery stalks, roughly chopped
- 3 garlic cloves, halved
- ¼ cup green onions, chopped
- 2 tablespoons extra virgin olive oil
- 1 can premium full-fat coconut milk (14 fluid ounces/400ml)
- 1 can water (using coconut milk can)
- ¼ cup chickpeas, cooked
- 2 tablespoons cilantro stems, roughly chopped
- 4 teaspoons lemon juice, or to taste
- 2 teaspoons grated ginger, firmly packed
- 1 ½ teaspoons white vinegar
- 1 teaspoon Himalayan salt, or to taste
- ¾-1 teaspoon dried dill, or to taste
- ½ teaspoon ground cumin
- ½ teaspoon black pepper
- ¼ teaspoon curry powder
- ⅛ teaspoon garlic powder
- ⅛ teaspoon cinnamon

DIRECTIONS

Place the carrots, onion, celery, garlic and green onions in a large baking dish. Drizzle with the olive oil and stir to coat evenly. Bake in a preheated 315°F oven for 45 minutes. Before the vegetables are done baking, purée the rest of the ingredients with the water in a high-speed blender, using the coconut cream can to measure the water. Then add the roasted vegetables and purée again until smooth and creamy. Serve warm directly from the blender or refrigerate for a chilled soup. This freezes well and can be gently reheated for future quick meals (don't overheat).

VEGETABLE FLAX CRACKERS

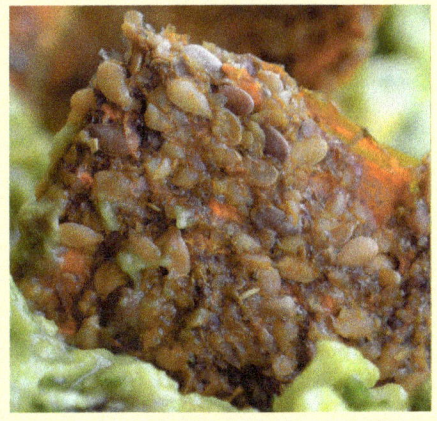

Calories	115
Protein	4g
CHO	8g
Fat	7g
Sugar	1g
Sodium	82mg
Fiber	8g
Chol	0mg

Per 10 2-inch crackers

During one of my stays at the Living Light Inn in Fort Bragg, California, I got the idea to experiment more with vegetable flax crackers. With all of the teachings about the importance of omega-3s, any opportunity to increase these in our home is welcome! My friend, Nikki Shattuck (one of the innkeepers), became my partner in crime—tasting and helping me brainstorm around the flavor-balancing and enhancement. Amazingly, the first go hit the mark. Unfortunately, I hadn't recorded any of the amounts, so a few days later, we repeated the process and were happy with the outcome: light, crispy, textured, and delicious crackers, which have endless possibilities for variation by experimenting with different herbs and spices. Have fun playing with this versatile cracker.

Makes about 25 servings

INGREDIENTS

- 2 cups carrots, roughly chopped
- 2 large red or orange bell peppers, deseeded and roughly chopped
- 3 cups ground flax
- 1 cup flax seeds (for texture and fiber)
- 2 teaspoons Italian seasoning, to taste
- ¾ teaspoon Himalayan salt, or to taste
- ⅜ teaspoon onion powder
- ¼-½ teaspoon cayenne pepper, to taste
- 3½ cups water
- ¼ cup lemon juice
- 2 tomatoes, roughly chopped
- ¾ - 1 cup basil (stems included), roughly chopped and packed
- 2½ teaspoons balsamic vinegar, or to taste

DIRECTIONS

Pulse the carrots in a food processor into small to very small pieces and put into a very large bowl. Without cleaning the food processor, process one of the peppers by pulsing in the same way and add to the bowl with the carrots. In another bowl, stir together the ground flax, flax seeds, and seasonings, then add to the carrot-pepper mixture, combining well. Process the water, lemon juice, tomatoes, remaining pepper, basil and vinegar in a blender until smooth. Stir into the flax-carrot-pepper mixture until completely combined. With an offset or other spatula, spread the mixture as thinly as possible onto 5-6 silicone-

(continued next page)

covered dehydrator trays. With a dull knife or offset spatula, score into small squares or triangles and dehydrate at 105°F for 12 hours. Carefully flip the crackers over onto the mesh dehydrator sheet, removing the silicone sheet. Dehydrate for 12 hours more, until crispy. Break into pieces and serve as a snack or side dish with soups, or as an appetizer with your favorite dips.

VANILLA ICE CREAM

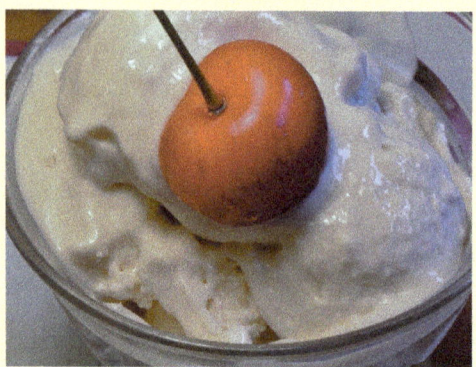

Calories	168
Protein	1g
CHO	15g
Fat	12g
Sugar	12g
Sodium	87mg
Fiber	1g
Chol	0mg

Makes about 2 ½ cups

Per ½ cup serving

INGREDIENTS

- 1 can premium full-fat coconut milk (13.5 fluid ounces/400 ml)
- ½ teaspoon chicory root inulin with Stevia or other favorite sweetener
- 4 large dates, pitted, to taste
- ½ teaspoon vanilla extract, vanilla powder or ½ vanilla bean
- ⅛ teaspoon Himalayan salt, or to taste
- pinch cardamom

A great treat for the sizzling summer month there is nothing better than cool delectab ice cream. This creamy vanilla treat could be easier to make, and with its low glycen sweetening, you can enjoy this pleasure gui free!

DIRECTIONS

In a blender, process all the ingredients until very creamy. If using the chilled canister type of ice cream maker, refrigerate the blended ingredients for 1-2 hours before processing for the best results. If you don't have an ice cream machine, use the Freezer-Stir Method.

Ice Cream Freezer-Stir Method (No Ice Cream Machine? No Problem!)

While more time intensive than an ice cream machine, the freezer-stir method can be used to make ice cream. Simply pour the blended mixture into a large bowl or flat pan and set in the freezer, stirring or whisking it every 15-20 minutes to break up the crystals until it reaches your desired consistency.

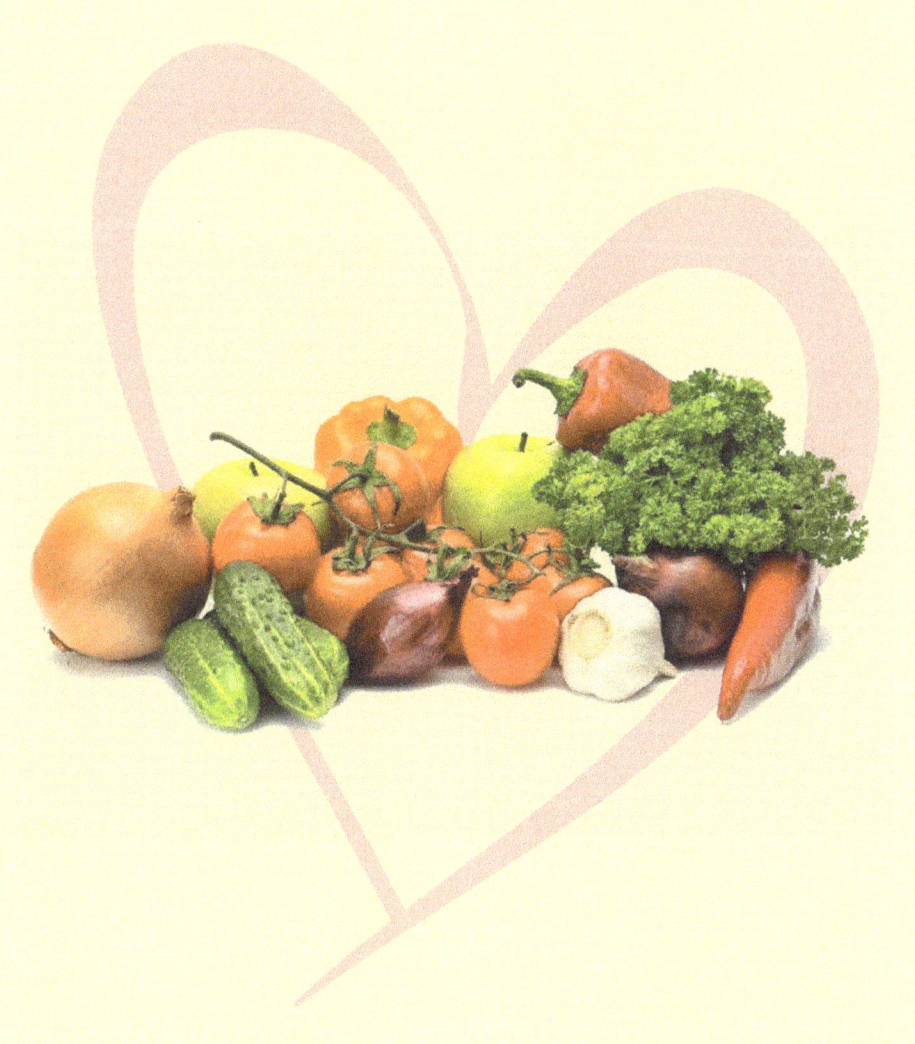

SUGAR CAUSED MY ILLNESS

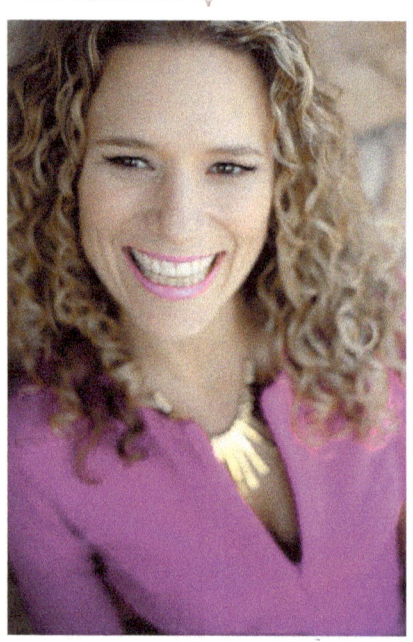

Stacey Morgenstern

I grew up in Philadelphia, the city of brotherly (and sisterly) love! I had quite the opposite upbringing from Carey (featured author, p. 58). I grew up on Mac and Cheese, Lipton Chicken Noodle Soup, Pringles, Ring Dings, Uncle Ben's Minute Rice, and a 24-piece bucket of finger-lickin' Kentucky Fried Chicken in the fridge at all times. The only junk "food" that was forbidden was Coca-Cola and any kind of taffy candy because "those are bad for your teeth." These early habits led me to be an absolute food addict in my early adult years—I was a compulsive eater and total sugar junkie.

I found a seemingly perfect fit for my love of sweets as a professional cookie and pie taster, and, yes, that's a job. But one day I was talking to a friend who thought that the culprit for my depression, lethargy, mood swings, and sluggishness was sugar—and that was my turning point. Once I realized this, I did everything in my power to change it because I'm the kind of person who thrives with a good challenge. Once I gave up the job and released being addicted to sugar, a whole new world of possibilities opened up that I could never have imagined in my wildest dreams.

The biggest step that I took to elevate my well-being was becoming a health coach. The way we teach it in our Become a Health Coach program requires you to look at your life on so many different levels, and this was my opportunity to assess and improve all areas of my life. I'm a personal growth geek, and that's one of the four pillars because you can't grow into the best coach you can be if you're not growing in your own personal life. This means pushing your edges and, yes, going beyond your comfort zone where the true magic happens.

What I love about health coaching is that it teaches you to trade in judgment for curiosity. I'm far from perfect; in fact, I don't believe in being "good" or "bad" with food. Nowadays, I eat delicious, nutritious, and whole food—meaning it grew either in the ground or on a tree, as well as some grass-fed red meat, wild fish, or organic, sustainably raised chicken. I also love to snack on yummy foods, but I do my best to stick to healthy snacks that boost my energy rather than deplete it. I eat for health, not just for taste. And even though I ate a ton of junk as a kid, I can be grateful that my body is so incredibly resilient and at forty-one I feel healthier than I was at twenty-one.

If you've ever believed the maxim "food is life," how about flipping it around to "life is food"? Because when your life is creative, your days are filled with purpose and meaning, and your relationships are healthy, your life feeds your soul. A great life begins, and sustains itself, with whole, nutrient-dense food.

When I think about my life now, and all that's transpired, I'm not so sure that I chose the path of a health coach as much as it chose me. I started to notice that because I looked healthy, was taking care of my body, practicing yoga, and eating good foods, people were constantly turning to me for advice about their own well-being. They were desperate, and I knew that with the right skills, I could help them achieve their best health. I'd like to share that you too can do this—it's not rocket science, believe me! The best thing about it is that the healthier you become, the more alive you will feel. And when you're truly alive, you are able to finally become the rock star of your own life, and there's nothing quite like it.

> Anything that looks like failure is simply feedback, and feedback helps you course correct in the direction of success.

Stacey Morgenstern

Founder of Health Coach Institute
www.healthcoachinstitute.com

BASIC STIR FRY

INGREDIENTS

- ¼ cup veggie broth*
- 1 pound of organic, free-range chicken (omit if doing vegetarian)
- 2 cups destemmed mushrooms
- 2 carrots, cut in matchsticks
- 1 teaspoon fresh ginger, grated
- 3 cups of kale, chopped
- ¼ teaspoon cayenne pepper (optional)
- Wheat-free tamari or salt, to taste

*SIMPLE VEGGIE BROTH INGREDIENTS

- 2 quarts filtered water
- 1 large onion, cut into 1-inch pieces
- 2 stalks celery, cut into 1-inch pieces
- 2 carrots, peeled and cut into 1-inch pieces
- 8 cloves garlic, crushed
- 2 bay leaves
- 1 large piece of kombu seaweed (optional, "the king of seaweed" adds great flavor; purchase at any health food store)

Calories	76
Protein	14g
CHO	3g
Fat	1g
Sugar	1g
Sodium	47mg
Fiber	1g
Chol	33mg

Per serving; serves 6

DIRECTIONS

Heat veggie broth in a nonstick skillet over medium high heat. Add meat if you're using it, mushrooms, carrots, and ginger. Cook for 5 minutes. Add remaining ingredients and cook until tender. Kale should still be green; do not overcook.

*To prepare veggie broth, add all ingredients to a large pot and simmer on low for one hour.

GENTLE LENTIL SOUP

INGREDIENTS

- 1 cup dried lentils
- 6 cups filtered water
- 1 strip wakame seaweed, cut into ½ inch pieces
- 1 onion, diced
- 2 cloves garlic, minced
- 1 carrot, sliced diagonally
- 1 parsnip, sliced diagonally
- 1 cup kale or spinach, loosely chopped
- 3 tablespoons brown rice or garbanzo miso

Calories	177
Protein	12g
CHO	33g
Fat	1g
Sugar	5g
Sodium	331mg
Fiber	11g
Chol	0mg

Per serving; serves 6

DIRECTIONS

Layer lentils, wakame (purchase at any health food store), onion, garlic, carrot, and parsnip in a pot. Pour in the water, bring to a boil, and simmer for 45 minutes. Add greens and simmer for another 5 minutes. Dissolve miso into soup just before serving.

MY BINGE EATING DISORDER WAS KILLING ME

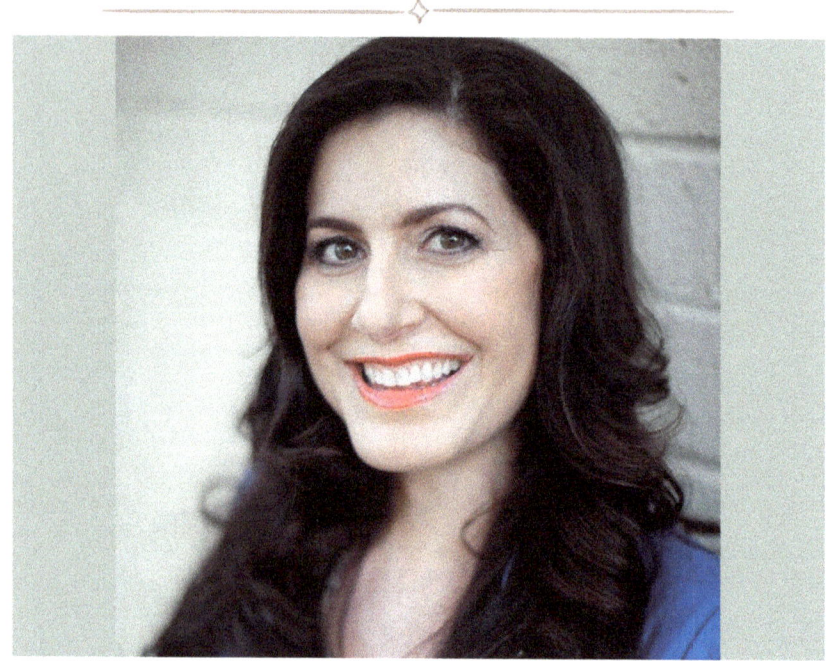

Carey Peters

I grew up in Birmingham, Michigan, a suburb of Detroit. My mom was a great influence in my life and one of her gifts was to make our food from scratch and feed us healthy meals. However, I remember whining and crying when she made homemade mac and cheese because I wanted Kraft! Despite my mom's attempts to set the stage for healthy eating, I had a 12- to 15-year derailment into the world of Diet Coke and processed junk food—like boxes of mac and cheese and a nightly tub of ice cream as a young adult. I was a sugar addict second to none, practically living on two liters of diet coke a day. This was really my life, and I was heading for disaster. I had an undiagnosed binge eating disorder and totally hated my life and myself. I was miserable.

Then one day I heard the calling. It was a little voice, a whisper, inside my head that said, "Come on, Carey, you're better than this! You deserve more from life. There is another way." I started admitting to myself that I had a binge eating disorder that was slowly killing me; just admitting that alone had an enormous impact on my health. I wish I could say that I went cold turkey and quit those bad habits overnight, but instead I entered into a gradual transition phase.

In my search on how to get healthy, I discovered that there was someone called a health coach who could help! It was not only a path that was significant in helping me personally, but I discovered an interest in becoming a health coach myself, as I knew that others faced similar challenges that I did. I didn't want anyone to have to face the same struggles that I had, and I believe that health coaching saved my life. Although it was hard work at times, I knew if I was ever going to be a happy person again, I would have to make some changes, and that started with my health.

Currently I am a new mom, business owner, and teacher, which leaves few hours for spending time in the kitchen cooking. So to help me out and to be at my best in all that I do, I have chosen to preorder my meals from a fabulous organic place here in Chicago. I'm a huge believer in outsourcing, so that's how I have solved my challenge of preparing nutritious meals. This company makes the most nourishing meals that would take me hours, even days, to prepare myself. The meals include full leafy greens, colorful veggies, delicious herbs, healthy grains, grass-fed protein, and it's delivered fresh and hot straight to my house.

Making these changes to my overall diet and lifestyle has had a huge impact on my life. The choices I have made set the necessary framework for everything I do as a health coach. It also helps to put me in a positive mindset, an uplifted mood, a creative headspace, and an open heart to the service I provide to the world. You can't really live, in the true sense of the word, without healthy foods—it is literally the energy that fuels your life.

While we often start a health journey by addressing food and what we're eating, it extends far beyond that—it also includes how we eat, why we eat, and where we eat. We teach these different aspects in the nutrition pillars for our Become a Health Coach Certification Program, as we find it's essential to creating optimal healthy eating habits.

Living on junk food is like trying to live your best life while your body is literally being poisoned. It's counterproductive, to say the least, which is why eating a fresh, nutritious diet is the surest and fastest way to a healthier, happier you. I understand the health challenges, as I have experienced them firsthand, and I also know from experience that there is a better way to live with health and happiness. I found the way and so can you!

> We can never in our wildest dreams imagine what will happen when we say yes to ourselves.

Carey Peters

Founder of Health Coach Institute
www.healthcoachinstitute.com

THAI SQUASH STEW

INGREDIENTS

- 2 medium leeks (white parts only)
- 2 tablespoons olive oil
- 2 garlic cloves, finely chopped
- 2 Serrano chilis, deseeded and minced
- 1 tablespoon fresh ginger, finely chopped
- 1 tablespoon curry powder
- 1 can unsweetened coconut milk (15 fluid ounces)
- 4 cups butternut squash, deseeded, peeled, and cubed
- salt or wheat-free tamari to taste
- juice of 1 lime

Calories	208
Protein	2g
CHO	18g
Fat	15g
Sugar	4g
Sodium	32mg
Fiber	3g
Chol	0mg

Per serving; serves 6

DIRECTIONS

Wash the leeks well and cut off the green parts, chop coursely into half-moons. Heat the oil in a wide soup pot. Add the leeks and cook over fairly high heat, stirring frequently until partially softened, about 3 minutes. Add the garlic, most of the chiles and ginger, and cook 1 minute more. Add the curry and tamari. Reduce the heat to medium, and add 3 cups water, coconut milk, squash, and 1 teaspoon salt. Bring to a boil. Then lower the heat and simmer, covered for 15 minutes or until the squash melts in your mouth. Add the lime juice and salt if desired.

SUPER VEGGIE SOUP

INGREDIENTS

- 2 yellow onions
- 2 green onions
- 3 celery stalks
- 3 carrots
- 2 zucchini
- 4 garlic cloves, pressed
- 3 kale leaves
- 2 cups broccoli florets
- 1 bulb fennel
- ½ bunch Italian parsley
- ½ bunch cilantro
- 1 tablespoon olive oil
- 4 cups low-sodium veggie broth

Calories	140
Protein	5g
CHO	19g
Fat	3g
Sugar	8g
Sodium	194mg
Fiber	7g
Chol	0mg

Per serving; serves 6

DIRECTIONS

Roughly chop veggies into small pieces. In a large pot, sauté onion, green onions, celery, carrots, fennel, zucchini and garlic in oil 5 minutes. Add veggie stock and bring to a boil, simmer, covered for another 5 minutes. Stir in broccoli for 3 minutes. Add kale, parsley, and cilantro. Cover and remove from pot after 2 minutes. Serve warm and enjoy!

ROASTED SALMON WITH MANGO-STRAWBERRY SALSA

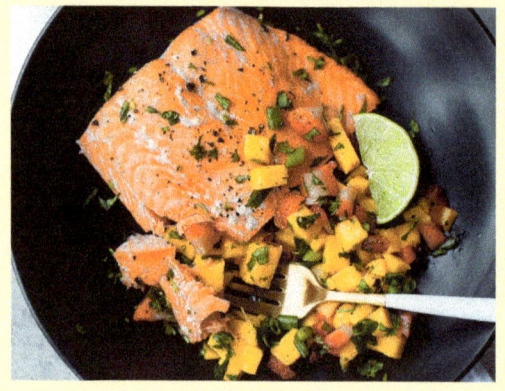

Per serving	
Calories	134
Protein	13g
CHO	4g
Fat	8g
Sugar	10g
Sodium	40mg
Fiber	4g
Chol	36mg

Makes 2 servings

INGREDIENTS

- 2 wild-caught Atlantic salmon filets (4 ounces each)
- Salt and pepper, to taste
- 1 ripe mango, diced
- ½ cup fresh strawberries, diced
- 2 green onions, sliced
- ¼ cup fresh cilantro, chopped
- juice of half lime
- additional lime wedges and cilantro, for garnish

DIRECTIONS

Preheat oven to 400°F. Line a small baking sheet with parchment paper and place the salmon filets skin-side-down onto the parchment. Season liberally with salt and pepper.

Roast in preheated oven for 10–12 minutes for a filet under 1" thick. You'll want to start checking for doneness around the 10-minute mark. You know the salmon is done when it looks opaque and flakes easily with a fork.

While the salmon is roasting, combine the diced mango, strawberries, green onions, cilantro, lime juice, and salt and pepper to taste in a medium mixing bowl. Toss to combine.

Serve salmon hot with salsa on the side. Garnish with additional lime wedges and chopped cilantro, if desired.

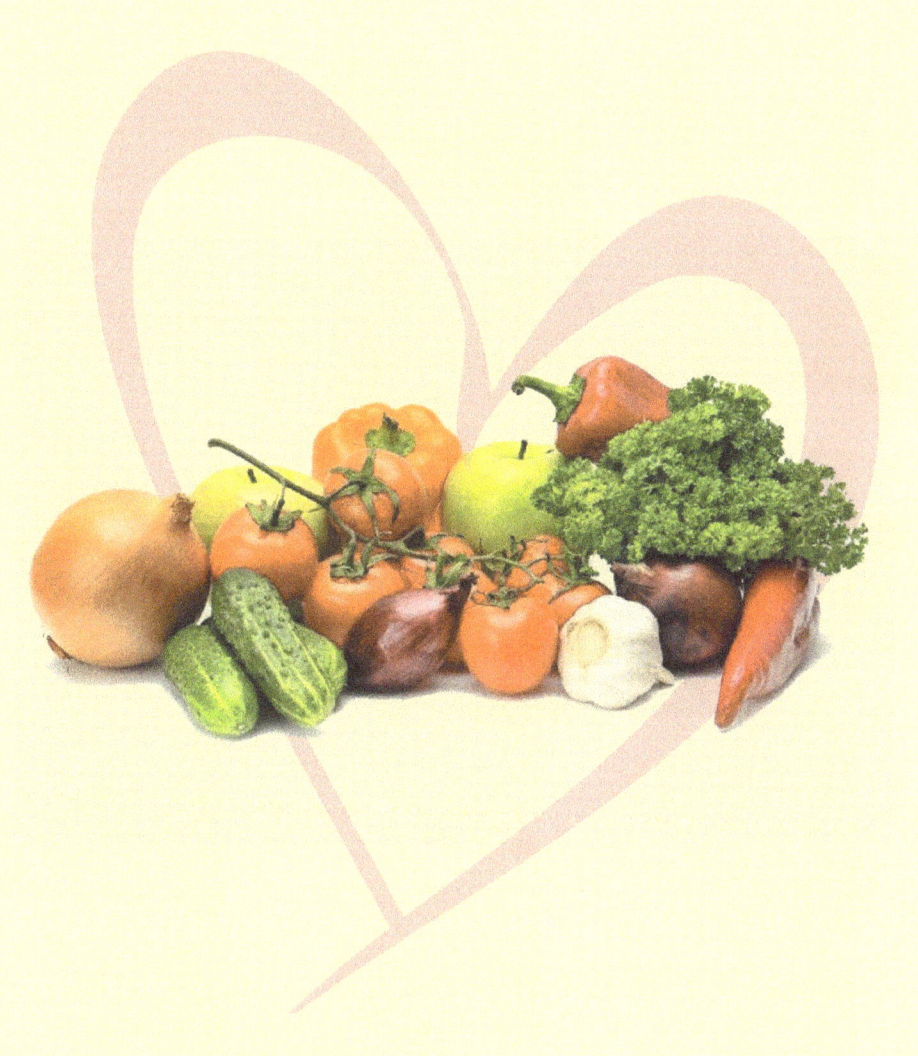

FROM FAT VEGAN TO SKINNY BITCH

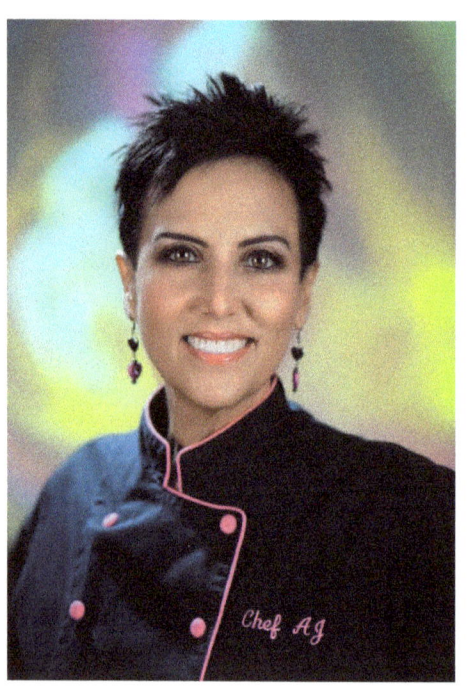

Chef AJ

My name is Abbie Jaye, but everyone calls me Chef AJ. I would like to share with you my personal story and tell you what I have learned about nutrition in a life that has often seemed to be food centered. What you eat affects all aspects of your being, probably more than anything else you do. What you eat has a profound effect on how you feel and look. Food can cause disease, or it can prevent and reverse it.

Unfortunately, I did not have this awareness for the first four decades of my life. I would now like to share it with you in the hope that you won't have to experience the same suffering I went through and watched my loved ones endure. Both of my parents died from preventable diseases (coronary heart disease and bowel obstruction) that were brought on by diet, and I nearly destroyed my health as well. It makes me angry, and it makes me determined to help others do better. Your diet can be your undoing or your salvation. The difference is the difference between processed and unprocessed food. I'm being generous in using the term "processed food." When there are no nutrients in a product, why do we even think of it as "food"?

What do I mean by unprocessed versus processed food? Whole foods found in the produce section or the bulk section of your grocery store or farmer's markets—found in the same state that they were harvested on a farm—are unprocessed; packaged food with a long list of ingredients is processed.

Now, I'm a vegan and I am passionate about recommending a vegan diet—a diet containing zero animal products—to everyone. It's better for your health, better for the environment, and better for animals. It's very possible to eat a lousy, junky vegan diet, full of oil and sweeteners and fake meats and highly processed grains. Those foods don't require animals to die, but they don't help you live in the best of health either.

I know that from experience. When I was a junior at the University of Pennsylvania, my anorexia became so severe and my weight was so low I was hospitalized for seven months, then transferred to a hospital in L.A. I was literally starving myself to death. Unfortunately, when I did start eating again, I didn't choose a plant-based, nutrient-rich, whole food diet. I choose crap, and my sugar addiction kicked into full gear. My nightly dinner became hot fudge sundaes. I gained sixty pounds, I purposely took up smoking cigarettes (thankful to stop just a few years later), I developed adult onset asthma and required much medication. I was then in a serious accident in which my spine was crushed, temporarily paralyzed, and was in a body cast for a year. I hit rock bottom, unable to live like that anymore. I turned to God. I began a spiritual practice that involved yoga and meditation. I also read a book that changed my life, *You Can Heal Your Life*, by Louise Hay.

For the first time in my life, I hit my knees and prayed to God. I remember saying, "Please just allow me to eat like a normal person and I will accept any weight you want me to be as long as I can easily maintain it without fasting, bingeing or over-exercising."

The entire emotional trauma I suffered took a toll on my diet and my health. My sugar addiction went through the roof. Instead of drugs and surgery, on July 6, 2003, I took another path that would change the course of my life forever. I used diet. I figured that if my food choices could either cause or at least greatly contribute to this disease, would it not be possible for better food choices to reverse it? I decided to go the "drastic route" and checked into the Optimum Health Institute (OHI) in San Diego, California. They taught classes that deal with healing on three levels: body, mind, and spirit. The most important education I got was mealtime. The diet was plant-based, organic, and 100 percent raw. The diet was free of what I have come to call "The Evil Trinity"—sugar, oil, and salt. Instead, it was based on fruits, vegetables, sprouts, and seed. On three of the days we did a juice fast, and I thought I was going to die. I would call my husband and sister every night and beg them to get me out of there. Like every addict, who eventually comes clean, I was going through severe withdrawal and detox. I complied with the program 100 percent. The abiding philosophy is that diseases occur when the body is in an acidic state and pretty much everything consumed on the standard American diet (meat, cheese, dairy, eggs, sugar, flour, caffeine, alcohol, oil, salt, processed food) serves to make us acidic.

We were taught that we need to alkalize our bodies, not by drinking some expensive water, but by eating fruits and vegetables in their raw state. When I got home from OHI, I felt better physically and emotionally than I had in my entire life. I was slimmer and looked healthier and younger. My skin was clear and my eyes sparkled. Six months later, I went for a follow-up sigmoidoscopy and my colon was completely clear! The doctors said it was remarkably clean this time, pink and vascular like a newborn's, and kept looking for the polyps to remove. They even accused me of going outside the HMO to get them removed! I told them that all I did was change my diet and they told me, "That's impossible!"

I knew that my addictions had eventually threatened my health and my life. And I knew that eating whole, raw, unprocessed food had done what my doctors believed was impossible, restoring my health and saving me from their interventions. A colonoscopy was done and the doctor said all was clear. Best of all, I did not have to come back for another ten years.

My dietary objective became, quite simply, to eat a whole food, plant-based diet with no added sugar, oil, or salt and absolutely no processed foods. Three weeks passed and, after being off processed sugar, my palate readjusted. Now, for the first time in my life, I could taste the sweetness in fruit and I loved it.

I am hoping by reading my life story, you may have had your interest pique about the many benefits of eating a whole food, plant-based diet, free of sugar, oil, and salt. My best advice to you is to just do something. Just because you can't do everything doesn't mean you shouldn't do anything. Optimum health exists on a continuum, and even small, incremental changes made consistently over time can still be of great benefit. You have to decide what your personal health goals are and how quickly you want to reach them. The first step in any journey is making the conscious decision to embark upon it. Then make a commitment that you will do this for at least thirty days. You really have two choices in life. You either commit to doing something or commit to your excuses about why you can't do something. I am giving you all the tools you need to succeed and to have boundless energy and health. You only have to ask yourself one question and answer it honestly: "How bad do you want it?" We all have dopamine receptors in our brains. Dopamine is a neurotransmitter that is released in our brain whenever we have a pleasurable experience. This could be having sex, taking illicit drugs, or even eating highly caloric food like a Big Mac, fries, and a coke. You can't just cut down on a substance you are addicted to and expect to regain your health. You need to quit. Remember, the only way out is through, there is a light at the end of the tunnel.

LOVING HEALTHY LIVING

Most people do not recognize the cause–effect relationship between diet and health. By the time you are diagnosed with cancer, it has been in your body for at least ten years. Just like a smoker does not get lung cancer from smoking cigarettes for a week or a month, the build-up of atherosclerotic plaque in your arteries occurs after years of eating a high fat, high cholesterol diet. Dr. Essenlstyn so eloquently says, "Heart disease need never exist, and if it exists, it need never progress."

About Chef AJ: Chef AJ has been devoted to a plant-based diet for almost forty years. She is the host of the television series Healthy Living with CHEF AJ, which airs on Foodie TV. With her comedy background, she has made appearances on The Tonight Show starring Johnny Carson, The Tonight Show with Jay Leno, The Late Show with David Letterman, and more. A chef, culinary instructor, and professional speaker, she is author of the popular book, *Unprocessed: How to Achieve Vibrant Health and Your Ideal Weight*, which chronicles her journey from a junk food vegan faced with a diagnosis of pre-cancerous polyps, to learning how to create foods that nourish and heal the body.

Based in Los Angeles, Chef AJ teaches a monthly sold-out seminar featuring cooking instruction, nutritional science, and song parodies, all delivered with comedic panache. Never content to leave her audience with mere "just do it" advice, she teaches how to create meals to transform their health, how to deal with cravings and food addiction, and addresses the emotional side of eating. She is the creator of the Ultimate Weight Loss Program, which has helped hundreds of people achieve the health and the body that they deserve.

Chef AJ was the Executive Pastry Chef at Santé Restaurant in Los Angeles where she was famous for her sugar, oil, salt, and gluten-free desserts that use the fruit, the whole fruit, and nothing but the whole fruit. Chef AJ is also creator of Healthy Taste of LA and the YouTube cooking show The Chef and the Dietitian, and is proud to say that her IQ is higher than her cholesterol. Chef AJ holds a certificate in Plant-Based Nutrition from Cornell University and is a member of the American College of Lifestyle Medicine.

> **If you aren't hungry enough to eat vegetables, you're not hungry.**

Chef AJ

Chef AJ - Abbie Jaye

TV Host of Healthy Living with Chef AJ
Author, *Unprocessed: How to Achieve Vibrant Health & Your Ideal Weight*
www.eatunprocessed.com

MINT JULEP DRINK

Makes 2 servings

INGREDIENTS

- 2 tablespoons lime juice
- 12 leaves of spinach
- 1 ounce of fresh mint, about 1 cup
- 2 frozen bananas
- 1 cup of ice

Calories	139
Protein	2g
CHO	38g
Fat	1g
Sugar	16g
Sodium	84mg
Fiber	10g
Chol	0mg

Per serving

DIRECTIONS

In a Vitamix or blender, blend the spinach, mint, and lime juice to a liquid. Add the remaining ingredients and serve. If you would like this sweeter, substitute unsweetened non-dairy milk for the lime juice.

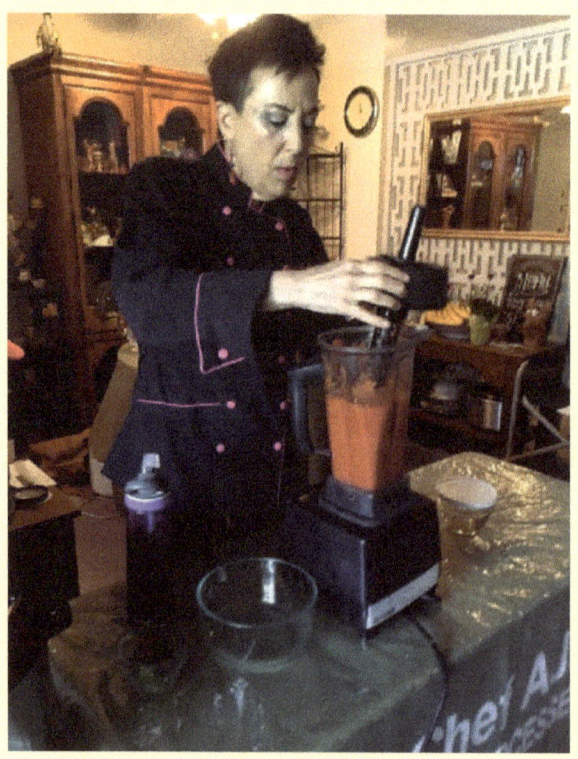

SWEET POTATO BISQUE

INGREDIENTS

- 1 ½ pounds of asparagus
- 6–8 large sweet potatoes, washed and diced
- 6 cups no sodium vegetable broth or water
- 1 large white onion, diced
- 8 cloves of garlic
- 2 tablespoons dried dill
- 2 tablespoons Benson's Table Tasty (or other no-salt substitute)
- 3–4 cups unsweetened non-dairy milk (depending on desired thickness)
- 4 tablespoons of low sodium Dijon or salt-free stone ground mustard
- 4 tablespoons of nutritional yeast (optional)

Calories	154
Protein	6g
CHO	43g
Fat	2g
Sugar	10g
Sodium	183mg
Fiber	7g
Chol	0mg

Per serving; serves 10

DIRECTIONS

Place all ingredients except for the non-dairy milk, mustard, and nutritional yeast, if using, in an Instant pot electric pressure cooker and cook on high pressure for 6 minutes. Release pressure and add the non-dairy milk, mustard, and nutritional yeast. Puree with an immersion blender right in the pot until smooth. If asparagus is not in season or too expensive, broccoli, cauliflower, or a combination of these vegetables may be used. Chef's Note: Delicious served over black, red, or wild rice.

CARIBBEAN MANGO SALSA

INGREDIENTS

- 2 (15 ounce) cans low sodium black beans, rinsed and drained
- 1 fresh mango, chopped
- ½ small red onion, finely diced
- 1 cucumber, peeled, seeded, and chopped
- 1 red bell pepper, deseeded and finely chopped
- 1 bunch cilantro leaves, chopped
- 1 bunch fresh mint, chopped (optional)
- 1 avocado, cubed (avocado)
- 2 limes (juice and zest)
- splash of orange juice
- pinch of cumin
- avocado halves or lettuce cups, for serving

Calories	154
Protein	7g
CHO	27g
Fat	3g
Sugar	7g
Sodium	100mg
Fiber	10g
Chol	0mg

Per serving; serves 8

DIRECTIONS

Mix all ingredients together. Chill. Serve in lettuce cups or avocado halves for a spectacular presentation. Chef's Note: If mango is out of season, substitute canned pineapple chunks in their own juice.

A TASTE OF SOUTHERN HOSPITALITY

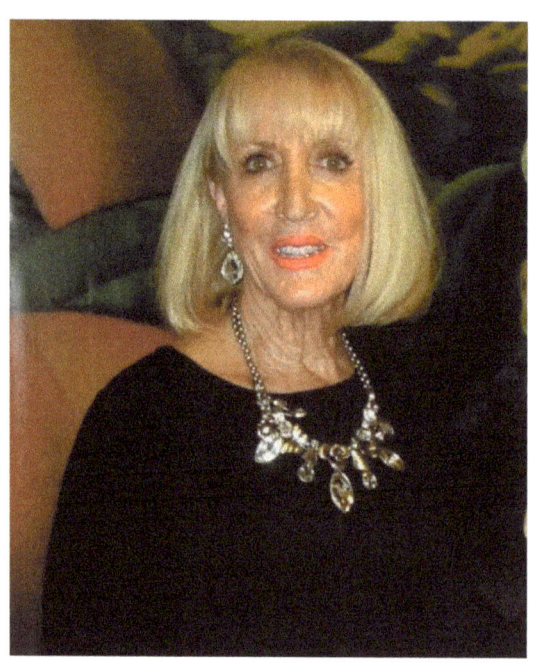

Martha Green

Learning to cook at the knees of my mother, I am often called the Inland Empire's Martha Stewart. I am renowned for my muss-free techniques and unique flavor profiles. You won't catch me recommending spun sugar or twenty-five-step recipes. While I am not afraid of food, I am an advocate for keeping things simple and letting each ingredient shine. A Southern gal at heart, I moved from South Carolina to the Redlands area in 1970. I have self published two books, *Martha Green's Cooking Things* and *Martha Green's Cooking Things 2*. I have served as the food editor for the Redlands Daily Facts, owned and operated cooking schools and kitchen stores in Redlands, Las Vegas, and San Bernardino. I have hosted local food-focused radio shows, regularly cooked for fundraising events, and taught cooking classes.

I spent time studying food in China and attended culinary schools in both Virginia and New York. Graduating from Le Cordon Bleu, I gained an appreciation for how the minor details make a big impact. Instilling my son JR with a similar love for cooking and food, we joined forces in 1996. Opening Dough'Lectibles, Redland's first scratch bakery, we made French delectables a favorite for many residents. We expanded our offerings with the addition of The Eating Room and Martha Green's Rustic Tea.

In 1994, I was approached by Redlands Bowl Associates. They were looking for ways to raise funds for the Redlands Bowl, and it seemed natural to raise funds for the bowl with its own cooking-school type class. I held cooking classes for over twenty years for the Redlands Bowl. I was inspired by the spirit of the entity I was helping, the vision of freedom and beauty known as the Redlands Bowl. Little did I know when first approached that I would lend a hand for twenty years, which another gal from the south had started the whole thing almost a hundred years before. Redlands Bowl visionary and founder, Grace Mullen, originally from Tennessee, often said that music is the universal language. I'd add, so is food; and you know in the South, we all think that a little storytelling makes the food taste better.

As I ended my last class of twenty years I decided to bring back the first three chairwomen to help, and to call the class "Curtain Call." While planning this, I also longed to leave a lasting good impression on the Bowl Associates—they have been so wonderful to work with—and thought the best way would be to compile all these recipes in a cookbook and donate half the proceeds from sales to the Redlands Bowl to help them in their mission to promote music and artistry in the community. I like to call this my "Thousand Dollar Cookbook."

For the first time, all together in one place, tasted and vetted by hundreds of good people over the years, they orchestrate my final curtain call as I bow out with my twentieth—and final—Redlands Bowl Associates Cooking class in 2013. Curtain Call recipes from all twenty years of Redlands Bowl cooking classes were dedicated to the Redlands Bowl Associates throughout time. There is a long line of compassionate people (I'm including the handsome husbands) intensely passionate about the original vision of Grace Mullen, who, in 1916, made available and free to all the best musical performance in a welcoming environment.

These women made me an honorary associate in 1996, and I found in working with them a very special quality of camaraderie, in which it has been a privilege to share. During this teamwork and commitment of twenty years, I have felt honored and blessed to have so many people come out to attend the classes year after year, to meet so many young enthusiastic women and men so willing to dedicate their energy to the community. Thousands of businesses have sponsored food and prizes for these classes as well. The Redlands Bowl seems to bring out the best in people; surrounded by such openness and generosity, I strove to make every class memorable. Over time, styles and cultures may change, but one thread seems to run throughout the history of Redlands Bowl—the belief that there is nothing that a community working together can't accomplish. I am happy to be part of that ideal continuing and through our era.

> "Wherever you go, there you are."

Martha Green

The Curtain Call Martha Green, Author
The Eating Room–Redlands, California
www.allmarthagreen.com

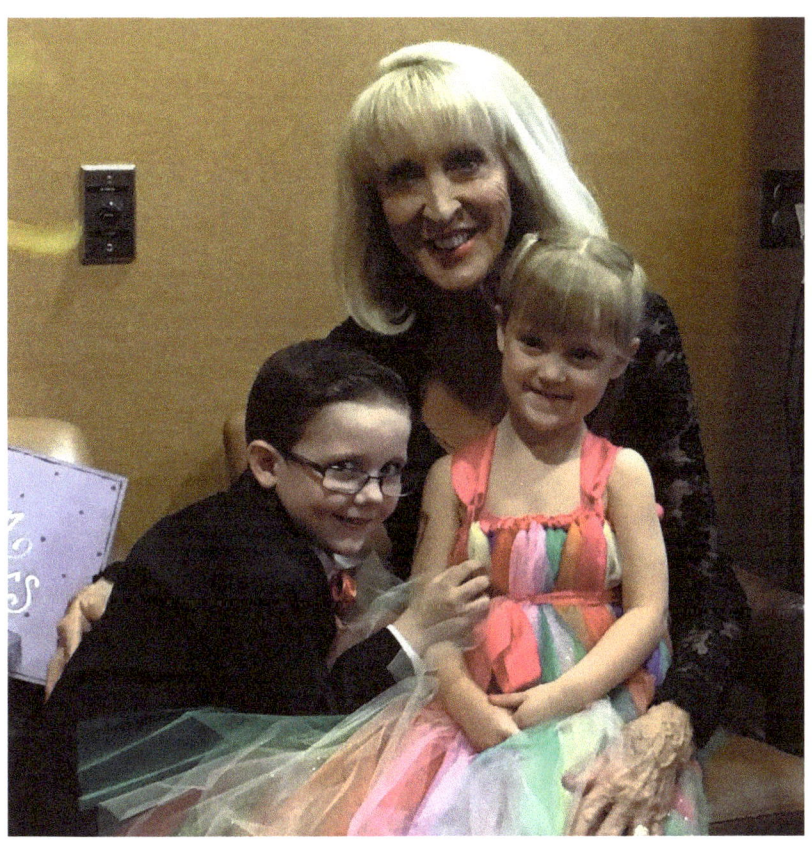

CHARLENE'S SULTRY SWEET CORN SOUP

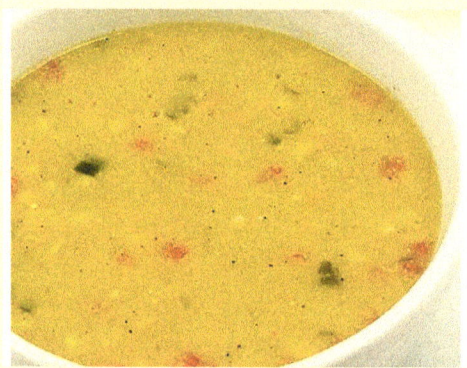

Calories	139
Protein	4g
CHO	17g
Fat	6g
Sugar	12g
Sodium	407mg
Fiber	4g
Chol	0mg

Serves 6

Per serving

INGREDIENTS

- 5 cups frozen sweet corn kernels (or 5 ears fresh corn sliced off the cob)
- 1 small red onion, coursely minced
- 2 teaspoons fresh Serrano chili, deseeded and minced
- 3 cups milk (non-dairy milk of choice)
- ½ cup warm vegetable broth
- 4–5 large basil leaves, cut in strips
- 2 teaspoons fresh lime juice
- 1 tablespoon olive oil
- 1 lime for garnish

DIRECTIONS

In a large pot over medium heat, sauté onion in 1 tablespoon of olive oil until softened, approximately 3–5 minutes. Add corn kernels and chili, stir to combine.

Add milk of choice and simmer, partially covered, about 15 minutes. Remove 2 cups of corn with a wide-slotted spoon and set aside. Puree remaining soup in a blender or food processor and return to pot.

Stir in reserved corn. Add warm broth to desired consistency. Stir cut basil into soup and reheat. Cut limes in half and squeeze for 2 teaspoons lime juice. Season soup to taste with salt, pepper, and lime juice.

THANKSGIVING MARVELOUS SWEET POTATO CARROT PUREE

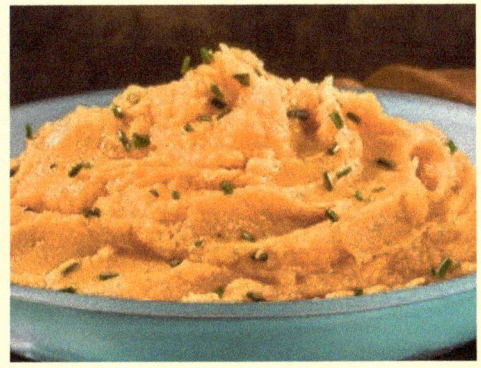

Calories	208
Protein	2g
CHO	28g
Fat	10g
Sugar	14g
Sodium	229mg
Fiber	3g
Chol	30mg

Serves 6   Per serving

INGREDIENTS

- 4 medium carrots, cut in round slices
- 2 large sweet potatoes, peeled and quartered (1 pound total)
- ¼ cup butter, softened
- ¼ cup brown sugar
- ¼ teaspoon salt
- ¼ teaspoon pepper
- 3–4 tablespoons whipping cream, light cream, or half and half

DIRECTIONS

In a large covered saucepan, cook carrots for 10 minutes in enough boiling water to cover carrots. Add sweet potatoes. Return to boiling, cover and cook about 30 minutes or until vegetables are very tender. Drain.

Preheat oven to 350°F. Transfer cooked carrots and sweet potatoes to a large mixing bowl and beat with an electric mixer until smooth. Add butter, salt, and pepper. Beat until combined. Then beat in enough cream or half and half until moistened.

If necessary, return to saucepan and heat through over low heat, stirring occasionally. Transfer to 1-quart casserole. Cover and chill until ready to bake (for up to 24 hours). Bake covered for about 45 minutes or until heated through.

A BRIGHT SIDE OF BAD HABITS

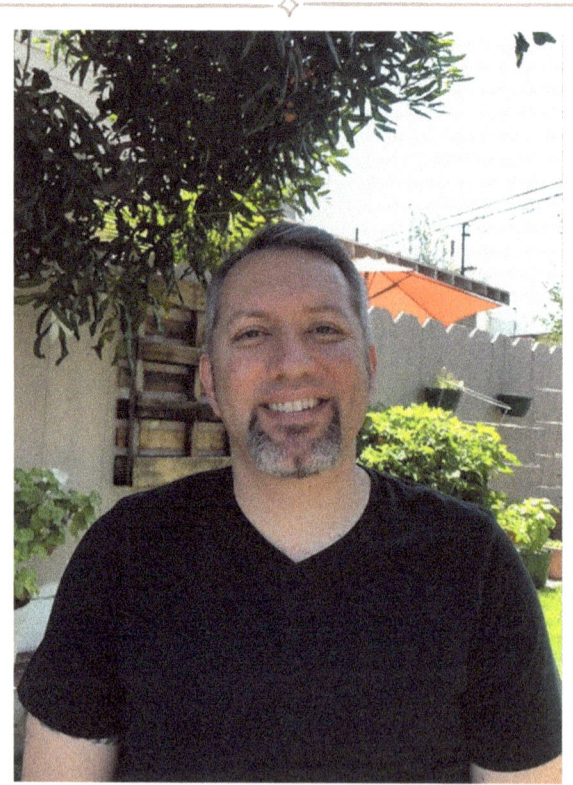

Chad Curtis

I grew up in a small town called Oroville in Northern California up until high school. At that time, my family moved to Sacramento and I finished school. Life was good, and I enjoyed a simple middle-class upbringing, going to school and playing sports. Dad worked while mom stayed home to raise the three kids. She made us breakfast every day before school, had a snack waiting when we got home, and dinner was ready by the time dad got home from work. We sat and ate together at the table as a family almost every night. We ate out at restaurants rarely. I grew up eating a typical American diet, which included the majority of vegetables coming from cans, a plethora of packaged foods, white bread and instant rice, and, of course, meat with every meal. I was fortunate enough to eat three meals a day and had all the food I needed.

I saw no immediate effects of those dietary habits as a child. I was active, and my weight was normal, with no apparent health issues. It was a slow decline over thirty-eight years, which picked up speed when I turned twenty-one. I discovered alcohol, the bar scene, and all the bad dietary habits that accompany that lifestyle. In 2011, at age thirty-eight, I was sixty pounds overweight and diagnosed with high blood pressure, high cholesterol, and alcoholic's fatty liver disease. I was an overworked aerospace professional during the week and partied like a rock star on the weekends. This lifestyle began to take its toll. I was burned out, my body seemed to ache from the inside, I had no energy, and felt like my life was imploding. During that fateful doctor's visit, after being hit with the news of my health conditions, I was prescribed blood pressure and cholesterol-lowering medication that I would need to take for the rest of my life. I was bewildered. I was thirty-eight years old! How did I get here?

As my doctor stood looking impatiently at her watch, I expressed a desire to discuss other options. You know, silly ones, like reversing my health issues instead of "managing" them with drugs. With a deadpan stare, she explained that a doctor's role wasn't to prevent health conditions, but to treat them … with medication. I knew I was on my own at this point, and I left the doctor's office frustrated and angry. This frustration soon transformed into a determination to heal my body on my own. I immediately cut out alcohol and became a vegetarian to reduce the load on my liver. Then, through a ton of research and effort, I made other significant lifestyle changes that produced dramatic results. I went back to the same doctor three months later for a checkup and my blood pressure, cholesterol, triglycerides, and liver enzymes were all normal and I had lost over thirty pounds. They are my lifestyle! As I continued to study, I discovered scientific-evidence-based, peer-reviewed studies and data that were not influenced by industry funding and quickly realized that what we are taught about nutrition was exactly wrong. I applied what I was learning to my own body and judged the results. My research eventually led me to what I believe is the healthiest eating lifestyle we can adopt, and that's a "Whole Food Plant Based" diet, also known as WFPB.

When I let my health get to the point of almost no return, I remember that feeling of shame, frustration, helplessness, and bewilderment. Although I was ready to take responsibility for where I was at with my health, I felt so overwhelmed I didn't know where to start. That's when I discovered a coach could be priceless. With someone providing support and accountability, my lifestyle changes were not only achieved, but also lasting. I had a deep sense of gratitude and wanted to give back in some way. I decided to give coaching a shot and never looked back. Being in corporate America my entire life, coaching was a completely new world for me. But it didn't take long to fall in love and realize this is what I wanted to do. This was how I was going to make a difference in the world!

The first and most important step was deciding that I was worth it! I realized that it wasn't about increasing longevity, as much as it was about the quality of my life. The quality of life now *and* later. The decision I was making in my thirties and forties was going to determine the quality of life in my fifties, sixties, seventies, and so on. The next important step was finally cutting out processed foods and meat all together. In 2016, I decided to follow the WFPB and cut out all animal-based products, along with processed foods. Really focusing on eating plants, legumes, and whole grains has been life changing. I've never been healthier. Most people don't realize that you can be a vegetarian or vegan and still be unhealthy. They're what I like to call "fast food vegetarians" who are non-meat eaters and whose diets consist mainly of cheese pizza, grilled cheese, pasta with marinara, potato chips, etc. Vegetarians who don't eat vegetables! This type of diet, although meatless, still does not equate to good health. Processed foods will negatively impact your health.

The other key decision was to start moving … consistently, everyday! With my eating habits dialed in, I began to feel so good and have so much energy I just naturally wanted to start moving. Not only am I working out, but I find that I walk, ride my bike, or skateboard almost everywhere now. I've picked up yoga to help with my flexibility, or lack thereof, from the weightlifting I do. With both diet and movement on track, I feel amazing. I feel better in my forties than I did in my twenties or thirties.

Being diagnosed with chronic health conditions and liver disease at thirty-eight was the turning point. It was the exact moment when I realized that I was slowing killing myself. For the first time, I contemplated my own mortality. I can't describe how it sincerely affected me, that by what I was choosing to put in my body, I was dramatically impacting my life. And the remaining life I did have would be filled with doctors, hospitals, painful treatments, and a ton of sorrow for my loved ones as they watched me deteriorate.

It finally struck me what "hard" really was. Was saying no to a cheeseburger hard or was chemotherapy harder? Was eating beans and brown rice hard or going through a liver transplant harder? Was eating a salad hard or having a heart attack harder? All of the sudden drinking my coffee black, cutting out meat, dairy, sugar, oils, salt, and processed foods seemed easy. It was a complete shift in my thinking.

Don't accept as fact that with age comes medications, limitations, and chronic health conditions. We all age, but this is about quality of life, and you alone control your quality of life as you age by what you decide to eat and the active or inactive lifestyle you choose. Decide that you are worth it, decide to love yourself, and take control of your health. Don't settle for managing chronic health conditions … eliminate them. You are powerful, so live the life you were meant to live!

As I said in the previous question, is eating fresh vegetables hard or is fighting cancer harder, or having a heart attack harder, or having a stroke harder, or having Alzheimer's harder? Think about it.

> I will not be discouraged
> with how far I have to go.
> Instead, I will be excited about
> where I'm headed.

Chad Curtis

Certified Health Coach
Long Beach, California
www.chadcurtiscoaching.com

DAN DAN ZOODLES

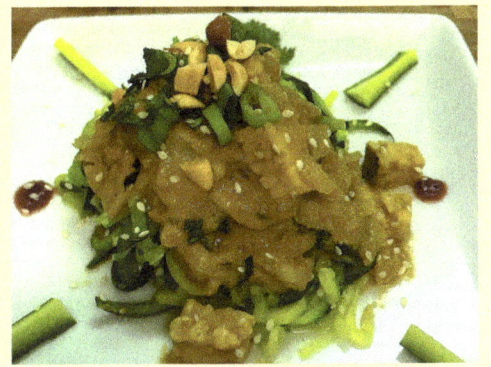

Calories	103
Protein	6g
CHO	7g
Fat	5g
Sugar	2g
Sodium	452mg
Fiber	3g
Chol	0mg

Per serving; serves 8

Inspired by a recent trip to Jose Andres' China Poblano restaurant in Las Vegas, where I devoured his Dan Dan Zoodles, I went to work in my own kitchen to develop a healthier version that we could all enjoy at home.

Out of all the recipes I researched, tried, and tweaked, the base of this recipe came from Chef/Owner Joanne Chang of Flour Bakery + Café and a Chinese restaurant called Myers + Chang in Boston. Chef Chang knocked it out of the park with this Dan Dan Zoodle recipe that was featured in *Food and Wine* magazine. I just modified it to make it a bit healthier by replacing the noodles with zoodles (zucchini noodles), swapping out the meat for tempeh and replacing the peanut oil with chickpea water. This recipe captures the flavors and essence of the original Dan Dan Zoodles and brings a nice level of spice for those who like it hot. Is it as good as China Poblano's Dan Dan noodles … uh, yeah. But please, you be the judge.

INGREDIENTS

- 1 package tempeh
- ½ medium white onion, finely diced
- 2 jalapeno peppers, deseeded and diced
- 2 garlic cloves, minced
- ½-inch slice of fresh ginger, peeled and chopped
- ⅓ cup liquid aminos
- ¾ cup chickpea water, drained from can
- 3 tablespoons unseasoned rice vinegar
- 2 tablespoons Sriracha chile sauce
- 6–12 drops, liquid Stevia
- ¼ cup raw unsalted shelled peanuts
- 2 teaspoons Asian sesame oil
- 4 zucchini for spiraling (Zoodles)
- garnish with cilantro, cucumber, sesame seeds, green onions, peanuts

DIRECTIONS

Sauté the white onion and tempeh in a large skillet over medium-high heat until translucent. While the onions and tempeh are cooking, add the jalapenos, garlic, ginger, liquid aminos, chickpea water, rice vinegar, sriracha chile sauce, stevia, peanuts and sesame oil to a blender and blend until smooth. Pour the sauce from the blender into the onions and tempeh mixture and heat through until well combined. Using a spiralizer, spiral the zucchini into zoodles. Sauté in a nonstick skillet for approximately 6-7 minutes or until they begin to release their water, but be careful not to overcook. Remove from the heat and place in a colander to drain while you finish the sauce. Place zoodles in a bowl or plate and top with the sauce. Garnish with cilantro, cucumber sticks, peanuts, and green onion. Mix together and enjoy.

O-REN ISHII'S MISO SOUP

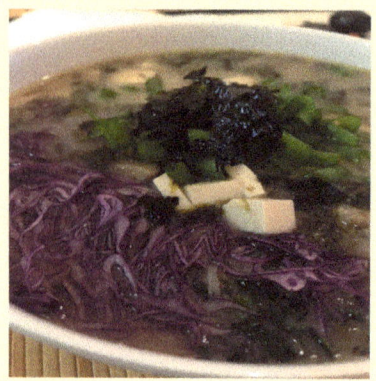

Calories	85
Protein	5g
CHO	12g
Fat	3g
Sugar	4g
Sodium	333mg
Fiber	3g
Chol	0mg

Per serving; serves 10

I've taken the often overlooked miso soup, haphazardly served at the beginning of a sushi dinner, and transformed it into the dinner itself. No longer forgotten, this miso soup shines like the rising sun on a crisp cold Tokyo morning.

INGREDIENTS

- 1 package of mushrooms (8 ounces), sliced
- 1 medium white onion, finely diced
- 1 quart water
- ¼ red cabbage, thinly sliced with a mandolin
- 12 ounces tofu
- ½ red onion, thinly sliced with a mandolin
- green onions, diced
- ½ cup dried seaweed snack (nori)
- 6 tablespoons low-sodium white miso paste
- 4 ounces thin noodles (optional)

DIRECTIONS

Sauté mushrooms and white onion in a 4 quart pot over medium-high heat until translucent, approximately 5 minutes. Add the water and bring to a boil. When boiling, reduce the heat to medium and then remove 2 cups of water from the pot and mix with the miso paste, using a whisk until smooth. Add tofu and ¾ of the dried seaweed (save the rest for garnishing) to the pot. If using noodles, cook them in the soup for the recommended time on the package. When noodles are done, turn off the heat and add the miso paste mixture back to the pot. Stir to combine.

To assemble the bowl, place cabbage, red onion in the bottom and fill with soup. Garnish with sliced green onions and the remaining dried seaweed.

Chef's note: I like mine spicy, so I add some sriracha hot chili sauce to my bowl.

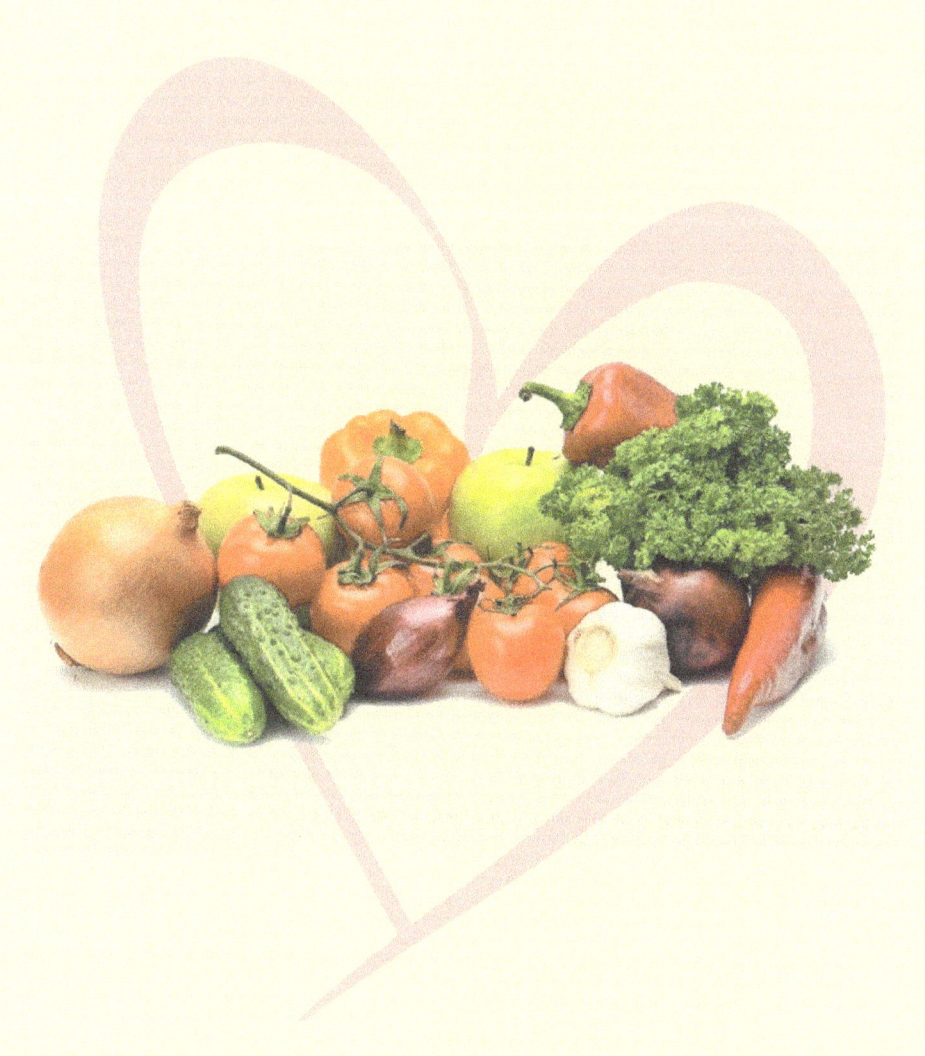

MY JOURNEY WITH GUT HEALTH

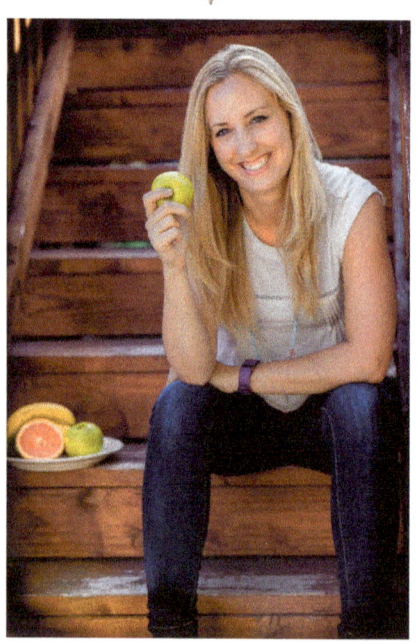

Tina Jordan Amoah

I was born and raised in the north of Germany, where so called "healthy meals" were common place. My grandparents had a garden where they grew a lot of organic vegetables. I never really wondered if food has a huge impact on our health until I moved to the United States to be an au pair fourteen years ago.

My digestion was always good up until then. I tried many different foods during the eighteen months I lived in Connecticut and gained weight quickly, always feeling hungry. My hair was dull and my skin inflamed with acne. After I returned to Germany, it took me about one year to lose the extra weight just by eating the same way I did before I left. My digestive issues started to really bother me at that point. I started to research about digestion and visited different doctors and specialists. They did many tests and told me that I had IBS (Irritable Bowel Syndrome). One sentence that one of the doctors said really stuck with me after I did the colonoscopy: "Your body is inflamed inside, but there is no cancer." *How comforting*, I thought.

My beloved grandfather had just passed from colon cancer before I left to the US, and my grandma had it a couple years later. They ate a diet that included lots of meat, vegetables, dairy, and sugar (she makes the best cakes). Overall they were considered healthy. I was always interested in health but really started to read up on different topics when no doctor could tell me what was wrong with me.

I lived with the discomfort for over ten years and tried countless diets, detoxes, and pills. Nothing worked. I was eating vegetarian since shortly after I returned to Germany and overall felt much healthier. But the issues were still present. Then I went to an alternative health practitioner, and she said I had candida, an overgrowth of bad bacteria in the gut. As well, I had aluminum and Teflon in my body, which explained the constant headaches. After the six-month treatment with the zapper, natural pills, and colon hydro therapy, I was like new. All my issues had vanished. Since that period, I have managed to maintain good health and increased my well-being more and more.

Today I incorporate a lot more greens, super foods, fermented foods (prebiotics) into my diet. I use anti-inflammatory spices and plants whenever I can. I drink more water, move more, and most importantly am a lot less stressed and worried. I started to love and accept myself and have finally cleared up my acne as a result of these changes. It has been a long journey but definitely worth it!

LOVING HEALTHY LIVING

> *Take care of your body; it is the only place you have to live!*

Jim Rohn

Tina Jordan-Amoah

Certified Holistic Health Coach
Long Beach, California
www.gutfeelingla.com
email@gutfeelingla.com

HEALTHY LEFTOVER MEAL

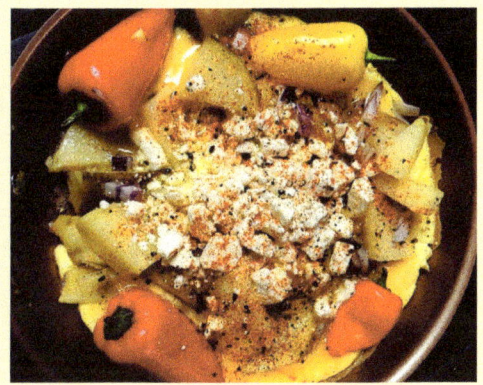

Calories	197
Protein	9g
CHO	29g
Fat	5g
Sugar	7g
Sodium	175mg
Fiber	4g
Chol	13mg

Serves 2   Per serving

INGREDIENTS

- 2 sweet potatoes, peeled and cubed
- 1 tablespoon olive oil
- ½ green pepper and ½ red pepper, seeded and diced
- 3 egg whites
- ¼ cup red onions, diced
- ½ teaspoon turmeric
- ½ teaspoon nutmeg
- pinch of Himalayan sea salt
- black pepper, to taste
- ¼ cup feta cheese, for garnish

DIRECTIONS

Boil sweet potatoes until slightly softened, then drain. Add olive oil to medium heat pan and sauté sweet potato with the chopped red onions. Next, add mini bell peppers and let it cook for about 10–15 minutes. Then beat 3 egg whites, add all spices, and pour over the sweet potatoes.

Lower the temperature and let it cook for a few minutes. Top with feta cheese.

PASTA WITH PESTO & FIGS

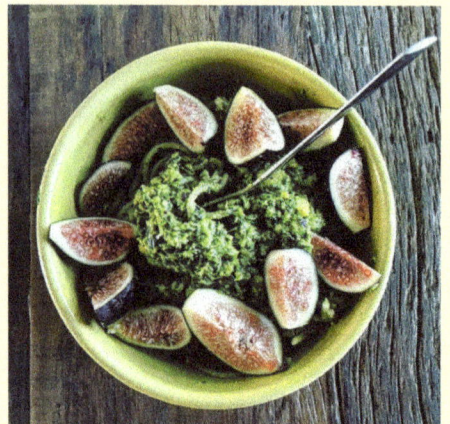

Calories	209
Protein	3g
CHO	15g
Fat	16g
Sugar	3g
Sodium	39mg
Fiber	2g
Chol	0mg

Serves 4

Per serving

INGREDIENTS

- 2 pounds spaghetti (made with brown rice and quinoa)
- ½ cup raw walnuts, chopped
- 2 cups fresh basil
- 1 tablespoon nutritional yeast
- 2 small garlic cloves
- 4 teaspoons freshly squeezed lemon juice
- ¼ teaspoon lemon zest (optional but recommended)
- ¼ teaspoon salt, to taste
- ½ cup olive oil
- 3 figs

DIRECTIONS

Boil the spaghetti al dente, according to the instructions on the package, and set aside when done.

For the pesto, pulse the walnuts in a food processor until broken into small pieces. Add the rest of the ingredients, except for olive oil and figs, and pulse a few more times until the ingredients are combined. Scrape the sides to incorporate any large pieces that remain, if needed. With the processor running, add the olive oil in a thin stream and continue to blend until fully incorporated. Stop to scrape the sides if needed and continue blending until the pesto is smooth. Season with salt to taste.

Mix the spaghetti and the pesto in a bowl. Then slice the fresh figs into wedges and place them on top as garnish. If you like, add some grated Parmesan and enjoy!

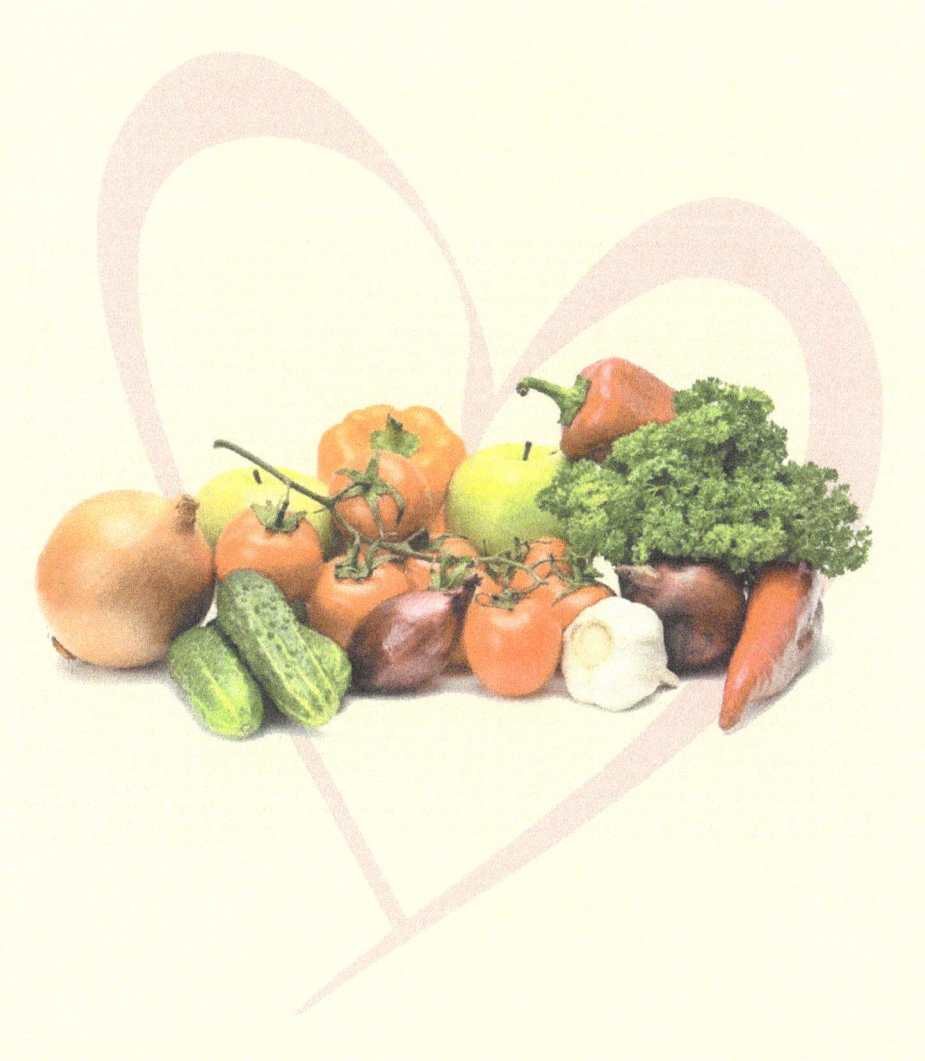

RAISING VOICES, LIFTING SPIRITS, CHANGING LIVES

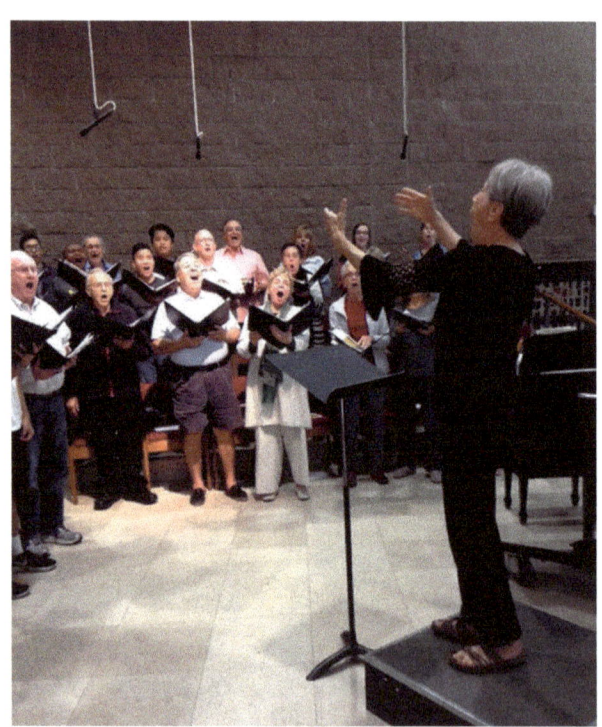

Meg Zeleny

Since 1981, Margaret Zeleny has been conductor and artistic director of the critically acclaimed Pasadena Repertory Singers—now the Downey Master Chorale, parent organization to the Downey Youth Chorale. In 1985, she founded the California Children's Choir with the sponsorship of the R.D. Colburn School of Performing Arts and the Pasadena Conservatory. The program she created for them is the model for DYC. Now sponsored by the Cornerstone Christian Worship Center, she brings the same quality program to Downey and its environs.

As a professional, she combines performing with educative skills seasoned with years of teaching junior high through college level, the fruit of which is a unique ability to communicate in both rehearsal and concert. Composers seek her out to premiere their works. Orchestras appreciate her clarity and architectural sense. Choirs look upon her rehearsals as group voice lessons. She leaves no one indifferent. All is done with a joy and wonder. She has performed in ten languages and can coach seven of them. Equally schooled in and comfortable with opera, musical theater, church music, oratorio, art songs, ballads, jazz, pop, rock, she has been featured as soloist with such diverse organizations as New York City Opera, Pacific Opera Theater, Carmel Bach Festival, Oregon Bach Festival, Los Angeles Master Chorale, Roger Wagner Chorale, William Hall Chorale, American Ballet Theater, LA Philharmonic, Beach Cities Symphony, Detroit, Omaha, Minnesota, Seattle and Dayton Orchestras, Les Brown and His Band of Renown, the Singing Sergeants of the Air Force, and Pink Floyd.

Margret has taught and conducted at the famed Interlochen Music Camp, the Angeles Oaks Music Camp Big Bear, Pasadena Conservatory of Music, R.D. Colburn School of Performing Arts in LA, at the Universities of Redlands, Iowa and Minnesota, at Whittier College, and Long Beach City College. She is a choral specialist and possesses a unique understanding of the young voice. Her groups are asked to perform in films, live radio broadcasts, and concert tours. They have recorded for Disney and have serenaded mayors and celebrities and archbishops. They have provided special music for weddings, funerals, anniversaries, dedications, and inner city schools where music programs are lacking.

Ms. Zeleny continues her work here in Southern California with young people in order to fill the void left from cuts in school funding for the arts. It is her intent that DYC reaches out as ambassador on behalf of the youth of the Southland. She was the first director of Loma Linda's Girls' Choir.

When asked how she maintains her health and youthfulness, she replied with an eager, "I Love Veggies! My best foodie memories are grazing on wild asparagus shoots and sprigs of anise in the dewy Minnesota spring mornings. Being a city girl, it was hard to find forage. Luckily, my uncle purchased three acres of an unused strip of land adjacent to a large cemetery where he set up a 'Victory Garden' (World War II practice in the 1940s during homefront food rationing). Daily, as we worked the fields, my brother and I could feast on carrots, celery, radishes, sweet peas, cherry tomatoes, kohlrabi, grapes, plums, apples, and cherries. Abundant were the fresh flavors enhanced by the warmth of the sun, all with no pesticides.

Minnesota winters left limited fare, but our cellar held sweet potatoes, parsnips, Yukon golds, and hardy apples for the lean months. Everything else had been neatly preserved in mason jars. I never saw an artichoke or avocado until I was thirty-seven. Small wonder that these days, my herbivore habits are served by local farmers' markets. I still do not eat much meat except, as in my youth, fish which we caught, and chicken which we bartered for. Perhaps all of this has left me, at eighty-three, still energetic and productive and prescription free. Must be my make-do upbringing, which, out of necessity, was so aligned with basics and the simple life.

By the time I turned eight, I was the family cake baker. Once you know the skill, it becomes an adventure modifying the recipe with switches and add-ons. I've included my favorite, carrot cake, in this book. It is also a sly way to get your daily fruits and veggies and essential oils."

Then she adds, "I am still conducting choirs, teaching voice and piano. I also enjoy walking fifteen to twenty miles a week and reaching out to those who need their souls touched."

> *Our greatest weakness lies in giving up. The most certain way to succeed is always to try just one more time.*

Thomas Alva Edison

Meg Zeleny

Choir Director
Downey, California
Email: mzmeg9@aol.com

CARROT CAKE

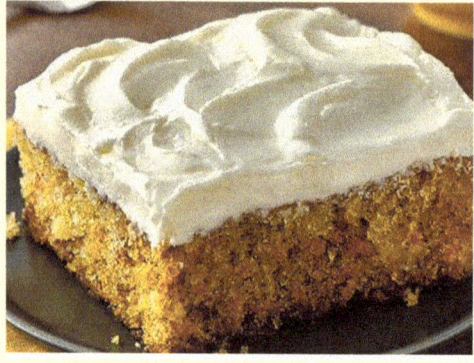

Calories	290
Protein	3g
CHO	42g
Fat	12g
Sugar	28g
Sodium	290mg
Fiber	1g
Chol	0mg

Serves 12

Per serving (does not include frosting)

INGREDIENTS

- 1 box carrot cake mix*
- ⅓ cup vegetable oil
- reserved pineapple juice
- ½ cup buttermilk
- 1 cup fresh carrots, shredded
- ½ cup shredded coconut
- ½ cup yellow raisins
- ½ cup crushed unsweetened pineapple, drained (reserve juice for liquids)
- ½ cup walnut pieces

*Note from authors: Boxed cake mixes are not ideal, but this incredible choir conductor, in her baby booming years, is still conducting and making a difference in people's lives. She desired to contribute this favorite recipe she has served many times.

DIRECTIONS

Preheat over to 350°F. Grease and flour 9-inch bundt pan. Combine cake mix, oil, and half of liquid (combined buttermilk and reserved pineapple juice) in a medium mixing bowl. Mix 2 minutes on medium or 2 minutes by hand vigorously.

Add carrots, coconut, raisins, pineapple, and walnuts. Combine well. Add the rest of liquid bit by bit to form a thoroughly moistened, but not runny, batter. If more liquid is needed, use buttermilk until the right consistency is achieved. Bake at 350°F until toothpick comes out clean. Cool completely and remove onto serving plate.

Frost with cream cheese frosting: Mix 8 ounces whipped cream cheese and ½ cup powdered sugar until creamy, then spread over cooled cake. Garnish with fresh coconut shreds or walnuts if desired.

GRANOLA

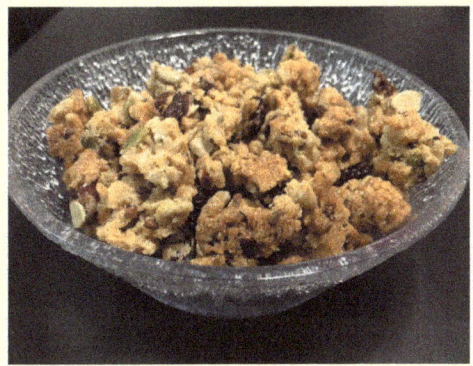

Calories	273
Protein	8g
CHO	31g
Fat	13g
Sugar	7g
Sodium	41mg
Fiber	5g
Chol	0mg

Makes 16 cups

Per ½ cup serving

INGREDIENTS

- 10 cups whole rolled or quick oats
- ½ cup unsweetened coconut, shredded
- 1 cup sliced almonds
- 2 cups wheat germ
- 1 cup raw sunflower seeds
- ½ cup brown sesame seeds
- ½ teaspoon salt (optional)
- 1 ½ tablespoons maple extract
- 1 cup water
- ⅔ cup olive oil
- ¾ cup maple syrup
- 1 cup raisins
- 1 cup dates, chopped

DIRECTIONS

Preheat oven to 350°F. In a large bowl, mix together whole rolled oats, unsweetened coconut, almonds, wheat germ, sunflower seeds, sesame seeds, and salt (if using). In small bowl, stir together maple extract, water, olive oil, and syrup. Pour over dry mixture. Mix very well.

Divide granola between two baking sheets and spread out evenly.

Bake at 350°F for approximately 40 minutes, or wait until golden brown. Stir every 10 minutes.

Remove granola from oven and cool. Mix in raisins and dates.

Store in an airtight container to retain freshness.

UNDERSTANDING FOOD SENSITIVITIES

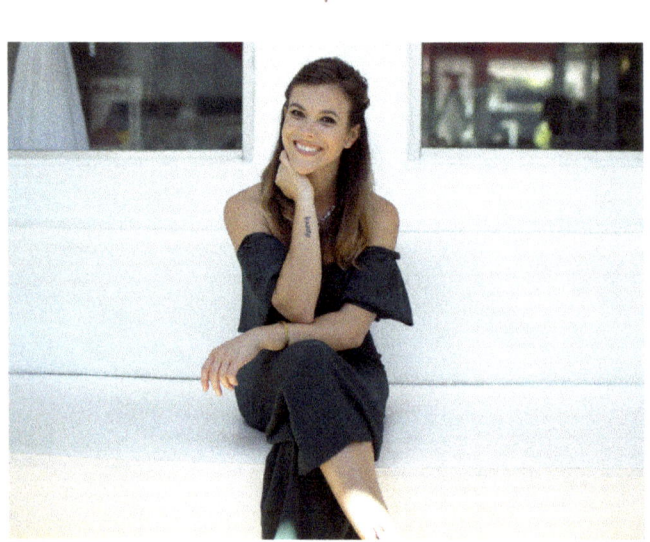

Samantha Schmuck

I grew up in Macomb, Michigan, as a very active young girl training in competitive gymnastics, which caused me to have a very large appetite! I can even remember eating as much as my brother who was seven years my senior. While I adored fruits and vegetables as a kid, I still had my fair share of processed foods, gluten, and dairy. I thought because I was so active I had the golden ticket to eat whatever I wanted, and I would be okay, making sure to limit candy as much as I could. I was never educated on how the body was affected by the different chemicals that showed up in our food system. I predominantly focused on how many calories I was consuming and burning, while ensuring I ate my daily fruit and vegetable quota. I continued in competitive gymnastics for about seven years, until one day at practice my wrists started to hurt and feel tender to touch. Soon after that, my shoulders were feeling the same pain, and then it was every major joint in my body.

After many doctor visits and multiple tests over the following year, the final words of advice from the doctor were to rest. All the tests were coming back negative; the only symptom was heavy inflammation, which all the supplements and shots could not reduce. I was a thirteen-year-old, stuck in middle school and feeling my awkwardness, when I had to walk away from my main identity in being a gymnast. Not once had my doctors ever thought to ask about my diet and the possible effects it was having on my body. For the following seven years I "rested," but the pain in my joints only lessened several degrees until I exercised then they would flare right back up again.

Although those years were quite dark for me as I suffered from serious bouts of depression, I wouldn't trade them for anything. I was able to learn so much about myself, discovered interests outside of gymnastics, and most importantly was led down the rabbit hole of health and wellness in hopes of healing myself. My real turning point came when I went to school at Life University to study chiropractic and found out that I was sensitive to gluten and allergic to dairy. I immediately noticed the brain fog, mood swings, and inflammation start to lessen as I cut them out of my diet completely. Nowadays I follow a gluten and dairy-free lifestyle consisting of mostly raw fruits and vegetables, nuts and seeds, lots of healthy fats, a small amount of animal protein, and very small amounts of processed foods. When I first cut out gluten and dairy, I panicked wondering what in the world I would eat. I knew an extensive amount about nutrition at the time, and yet that panic still washed over me. It was easy to focus on all the foods I had to remove from my diet, but then I was able to quickly shift and look at all the foods I could eat—that I had yet to experiment with.

It has been remarkable to see how my body has been able to heal itself over time when given the proper building blocks. As a result of my own health journey and learning how to improve my life, it was important for me to become a health coach and help others to become empowered in their own bodies again. There came a point where I felt like a stranger in my own skin, and the doctors who were supposed to have all the answers had none. As a health coach, I am able to help individuals reclaim their power and help them understand how they can live a vibrant and fully expressed life in all aspects, but that first starts by having a healthy body full of energy.

We all have our own reasons for eating a healthier, more nutritious diet that ranges from health concerns to simply wanting to be around longer for our loved ones. I constantly hear others say, "I only have ____ amount of years on this earth, and I want to enjoy my favorite things." I understand that frame of thinking, and yet there is a more empowered stance when you find all the joy and pleasure in the food that makes you feel unbelievably vibrant. This food allows you to think more clearly, have tremendous amounts of sustained energy, and feel absolutely sexy in your own skin—with endless possibilities.

Each day is a new day, with the choice to make today better than yesterday. You are your best experiment, and there is no better time than the present to take advantage of the abundant resources available to make a difference in your life today!

> Let us not hope for mere chance
> to change our story;
> let us summon the courage
> to change it ourselves.
>
> **Brendon Buchard**

Samantha Schmuck

CEO, Founder of Revived Living BS, HC
Certified Health Coach

BLACK BEAN CUPCAKES

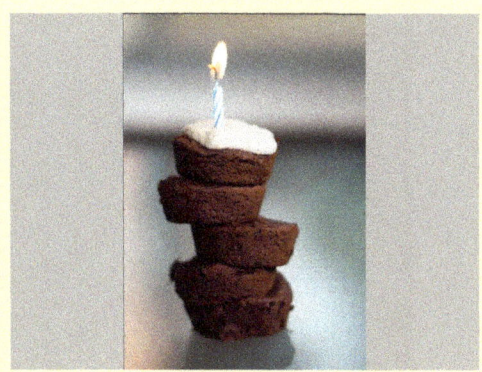

Makes 12 cupcakes

Calories	120
Protein	3g
CHO	17g
Fat	4g
Sugar	8g
Sodium	92mg
Fiber	8g
Chol	0mg

Per cupcake (does not include frosting)

INGREDIENTS

- 1 ¾ cup black beans, drained and rinsed (cooked or from a can)
- 3 tablespoons coconut oil (melted)
- ½ cup raw sugar (pulse it in the blender for less texture)
- 2 cheggs (aka, chia eggs, 2.5 tablespoons ground chia seeds to 6 tablespoons water*)
- ¾ cup raw cacao powder
- ¼ teaspoon salt
- 1 teaspoon vanilla extract
- 1 ½ teaspoons baking powder

DIRECTIONS

Preheat the oven to 350°F and grease a muffin pan with coconut oil and lightly flour.

*Create the chegg by blending the chia seeds until they are in a powder. Pour into a separate container, add water, and let sit while you prepare the rest.

Pulse the sugar until it is in a fine powder.

Add the rest of the ingredients.

Blend until a smooth consistency is reached, but be careful not to overblend it. You will most likely have to scrape down the sides several times. If it is too thick, just add 1–2 tablespoons of water and reblend.

Pour equal amounts of batter into the muffin tins and bake for 20–25 minutes.

Mine came out perfect at about 19 minutes, so just keep an eye on them. The edges will be pulled away from the sides of the tin, but the middle will still be a fudge-like consistency. (They are vegan, so no worries about raw batter!)

Pull out of the oven and let cool before pulling them out of the pan.

Chef's Note: The cupcakes are best when assembled right before eating; keep the frosting and berry compote (next page) separate until serving. These cupcakes are quite fantastic by themselves, with just the hazelnut frosting added, or with all three components.

HAZELNUT CREAM FROSTING

Makes 2 cups

INGREDIENTS

- 2 cups hazelnuts (soaked overnight or at least 2 hours)
- 1 ½ cups nut milk
- 1 teaspoon vanilla
- juice of 1 lemon
- 1 tablespoon maple syrup

Calories	51
Protein	1g
CHO	1g
Fat	4g
Sugar	1g
Sodium	8mg
Fiber	1g
Chol	0mg

Per tablespoon

DIRECTIONS

Place all ingredients in a blender. Blend until a smooth consistency is reached. Set frosting aside. Spread on the Black Bean Cupcakes just before serving.

MIXED BERRY GINGER COMPOTE

Makes 4 cups

INGREDIENTS

- 2 cups each: fresh blueberries, blackberries & raspberries (or 2 cups each of frozen)
- juice of 1 lemon
- 2 tablespoons raw sugar
- ½ inch fresh ginger, thinly sliced

Calories	34
Protein	1g
CHO	8g
Fat	0g
Sugar	5g
Sodium	0mg
Fiber	2g
Chol	0mg

Per 2 tablespoons

DIRECTIONS

Wash the berries and place all ingredients in a saucepan on medium heat.

Stir occasionally and, once the berries begin to soften, break them up slightly with a wooden spoon.

Continue cooking the berries approximately 20 minutes, or until the liquid thickens slightly.

Allow the compote to cool slightly, then assemble with cupcakes and hazelnut frosting when ready to serve.

ASIAN INSPIRED SALAD

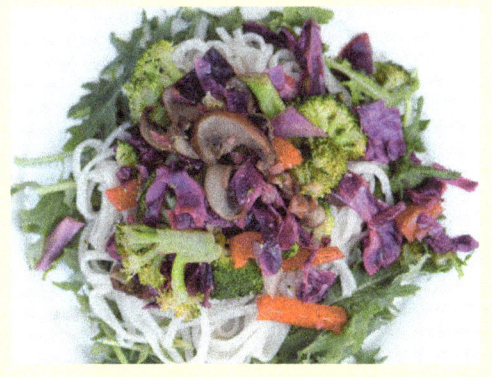

Calories	129
Protein	3g
CHO	19g
Fat	5g
Sugar	4g
Sodium	100mg
Fiber	3g
Chol	0mg

Per serving; serves 4

This is such a quick, light, filling, delicious, and, MOST importantly, beautiful dish that is sure to impress guests. This is a vegetarian dish, but you can certainly add a serving of protein as well.

Far too often we go through life throwing together our dinners or snacks, never giving a second thought to what it looks like on the plate first (except maybe when were are trying to impress a guest!).

I encourage you to try this: Take an extra minute and make your dish presentable, even if it's just for you! Digestion really begins with our eyes first, believe it or not, so it is very important to put together your dish with intention. Keep in mind: It does not have to be Martha Stewartesque (unless you want it to be). It can be as simple as using your favorite plate, or layering the different foods so the various colors and textures have a chance to shine on their own.

INGREDIENTS

- 2 tablespoons oil
- 2 cloves garlic, minced
- ½ medium white onion, sliced
- 1 cup mushrooms, sliced
- 1 red bell pepper, deseeded and chopped
- 1½ cups red cabbage, sliced
- 1 lime
- 1 cup kale
- 1 cup broccoli florets
- 4 ounces brown rice noodles, cooked
- 3 tablespoons of your favorite Asian style dressing

DIRECTIONS

Melt the oil in a medium sauté pan, over medium high heat.

In a separate pot, boil some water, and cook the noodles according to package instructions.

Add in the onions and mushrooms, season with salt & pepper to taste, and continue cooking until the onions become translucent, approximately 4 minutes.

Add in the chopped bell pepper, cabbage, garlic, and juice of the lime.

Once the vegetables have cooked to desired texture (I like mine more raw) add in the broccoli and cover with a lid. By adding the broccoli last and gently steaming it, you are able to keep the beautiful green color.

Last, stir in the dressing. I used a sweet and tangy Asian sesame dressing.

On a plate, lay a bed of kale and press down. Next, top with a helping of noodles, and finish it by topping with lots of vegetables. Here you can add more lime juice or just a wee bit of dressing if you would like.

I AM MY BEST FRIEND

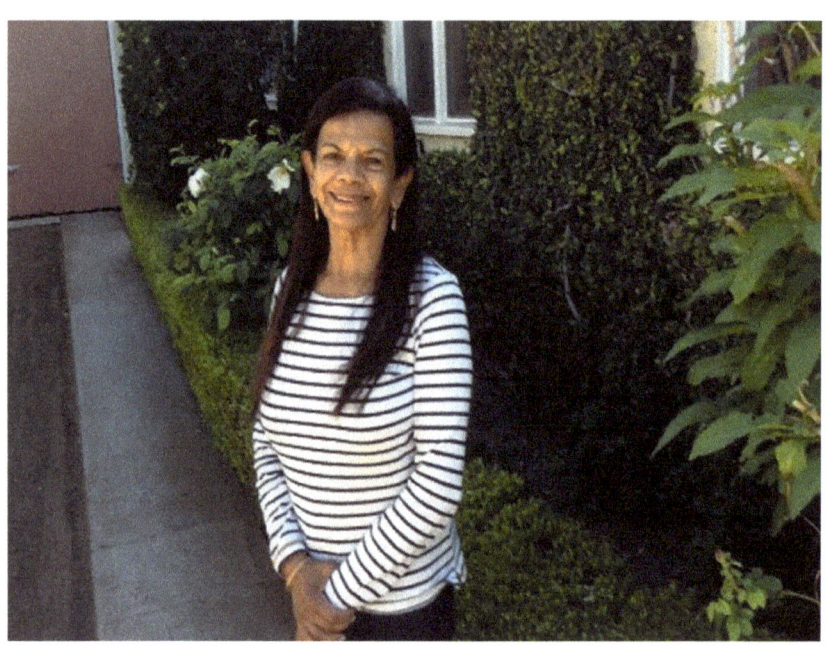

Bertha Noble

I was born in Sri Lanka, an island in the Indian Ocean. My childhood and most of my adult life was on the island, where living simply and eating food grown locally or in our home garden was the norm. The main items in our meals were seasonal food with fresh and plentiful fish, very little meat (meat was more expensive), vegetables, rice, and no packaged or prepared food. The primary source of carbohydrates was rice flour. Coconut milk was used in most of our food preparations. My grandmother was a vegetarian and stayed away from all animal protein, even eggs. Mangoes, pineapple, and all tropical fruits in season were also available as snacks and desserts. These simple eating habits never left me even though I came to England to further my studies. Graduating with a nursing degree, I moved to the U.S., where work, family, and the many stresses of life affected my health. Following many nutritional gurus, and reading nutritional research, I decided to carve out a path to wellness that fit my lifestyle and my beliefs.

Yoga saved my life, and the salvation has been stable and profound over time. It provided an instantaneous relief to focus on my palms and my feet. I started yoga in my midlife after an unfortunate and unwanted health setback that left me to re-evaluate my life, not just in my daily living but also to search my mind and my body. In searching, I discovered what I needed was a commitment to make changes without looking for results and to cultivate a life-changing path that would help me live my life to the fullest—with gratitude.

After eight years, I have discovered that exercise and simple food cooked at home is the answer to healthy living. I enjoy yoga to the fullest, as well as cooking meals at home, eating mostly vegetables and fish. I still eat meals outside of the home but stay close to my commitment to eat healthy. I also enjoy raw food whenever possible. Drinking my vegetable smoothie each morning leaves my body well-nourished and ready for the day. With my commitment to better health has come more emphasis on my faith, that God will do what is needed to bring my left and right brain in alignment. In yoga, I have learned that transitions between the postures are the measure of grace, as much as the postures themselves. Learning to settle in the moment continues to help me in my worship, in my relationships with my family, friends, and my yoga family. In this life-changing journey, I have learned I am my best friend.

I realize aging is inevitable for all of us, yet for so many I know it is a surprise. Some are not able to accept what it is. Yes, the physical experience in yoga has made me enjoy my gardening more than I ever imagined. But I made a decision to be more fascinated about the aging process than terrified. There is grief to be had, to be sure, and fear, and lots of simple disappointments, but settling into this as best as I am able, I experience an unexpected gift of contentment. Contentment is not something I ever really knew I wanted, but this too is God's grace. There is no experience more pleasurable than my first cup of tea in the morning, no view more breathtaking than the tall camphor tree that stands day in and day out in my back yard. I see beauty in acts of kindness, in humans reaching out to one another, and through this *Loving Healthy Living* book. May this kindness bring grace to visit someone's life, like it did mine.

> May you bloom whereever you are planted.

Bertha Noble

Registered Nurse
Redlands, California

ASIAN SALMON BOWL

Serves 2

INGREDIENTS

- 4 teaspoons rice vinegar
- ½ teaspoon grated ginger
- 1 teaspoons miso paste
- 2 teaspoons low sodium soy sauce
- 2 tablespoons vegetable oil
- 2 tablespoons toasted sesame oil
- 1 ½ cups cooked wild rice
- 6 ounces wild caught Atalntic salmon, prepared by your favorite method
- ½ cup frozen shelled edamame, thawed
- ½ cup carrots, shredded
- ½ cup snow peas
- 1large scallion, sliced
- ½ cup sesame seeds
- red pepper flakes, for garnish

Calories	250
Protein	13g
CHO	24g
Fat	12g
Sugar	3g
Sodium	150mg
Fiber	4g
Chol	45mg

per serving

DIRECTIONS

Whisk rice vinegar, ginger, miso, soy sauce, and 1 teaspoon warm water. Set aside. (Dressing is best when made ahead of time and refrigerated 4 hrs before serving.)

Divide cooked wild rice rice between 2 bowls and top each with prepared salmon, raw edamame, raw carrots and raw snow peas. Drizzle with dressing and top with scallion and sesame seeds. Garnish with red pepper flakes.

CASHEW AND PEPPER STIR-FRY

Serves 2

INGREDIENTS

- 3 teaspoons low sodium soy sauce
- 1 teaspoon seasoned rice vinegar
- 2 teaspoons cornstarch
- 2 teaspoons honey
- 2 teaspoons vegetable oil
- 2 cloves of garlic, minced
- ½ piece of ginger peeled and cut into matches
- 1 cup snap peas
- 1 large red bell pepper, deseeded and sliced
- 1 medium red onion, sliced into ½-inch wedges
- 6 teaspoons roasted cashews, for garnish
- sliced chives, for garnish

Calories	80
Protein	2g
CHO	9g
Fat	4g
Sugar	4g
Sodium	150mg
Fiber	4g
Chol	0mg

Per serving

DIRECTIONS

Combine soy sauce, vinegar, cornstarch, and honey. Heat oil in skillet, then add garlic and ginger. Cook until lightly browned, approximately 1 minute. Add peas, pepper, and onion. Cook, stirring occasionally, until crisp-tender, approximately 3 minutes. Add sauce mixture and cook until slightly thickened.

Serve warm, topped with cashews and chives.

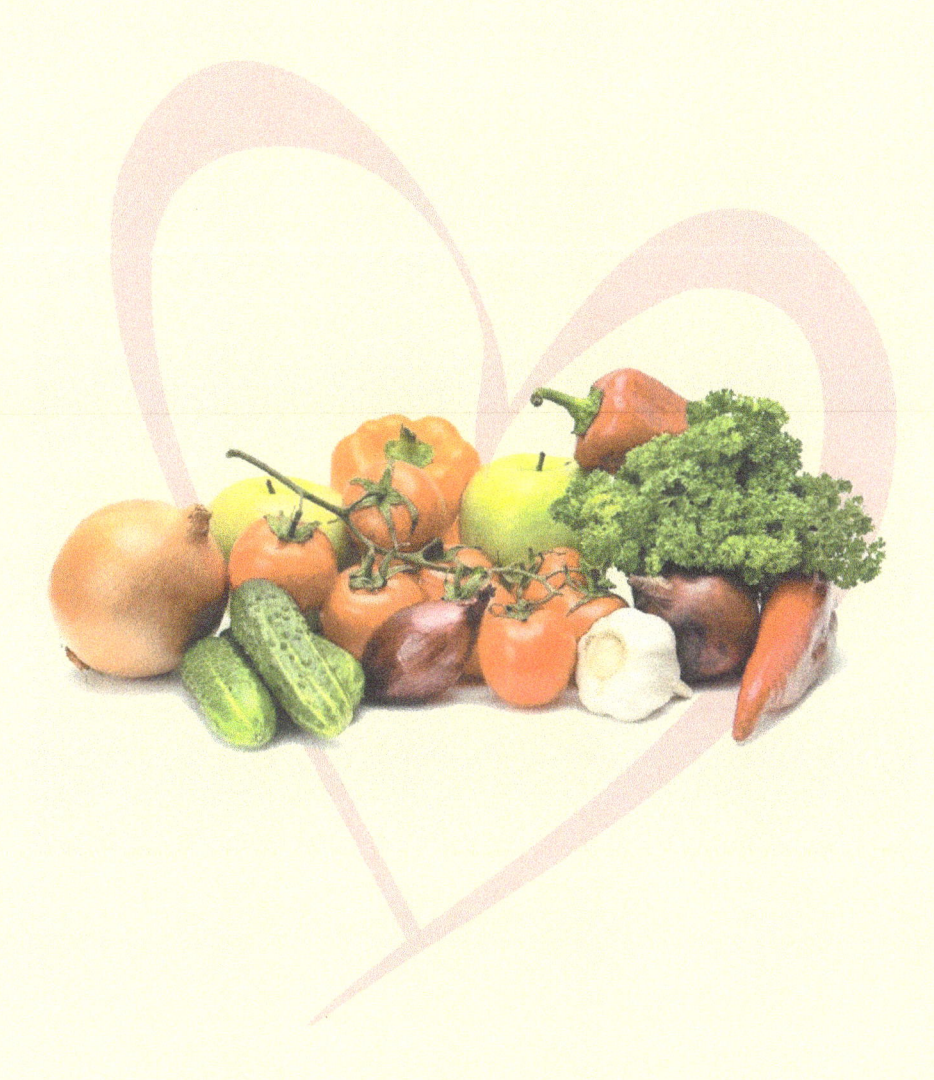

NOURISHING MY BODY & SOUL WAS LIFE CHANGING

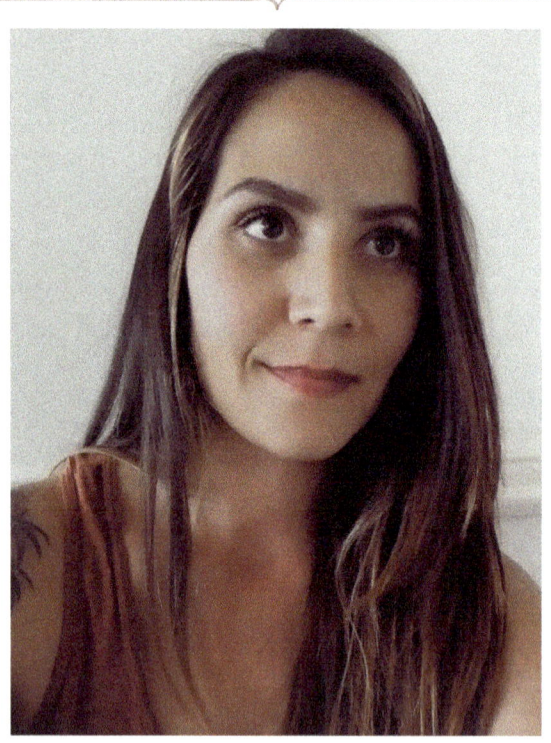

Nicole Jennifer Enns

I was born in Saskatchewan but lucky enough to grow up here on the beautiful West Coast of British Columbia, in a little beach city called White Rock. I say *lucky* because I would happily take rain over the snow, and I can't imagine living away from the ocean and mountains. Also, the lower mainland of British Columbia is very health conscious; there is no shortage of organic grocery shops, farmers markets, vegetarian restaurants, or yoga studios. It has been a wonderful place to grow up and has played an important role in my well-being today.

I am the oldest of three, and I grew up in a multicultural family. My mom is Filipino, and my dad is of German descent. To say that I have a large extended family would be an understatement. I have a dozen aunts and uncles and more than twenty first cousins who are more like siblings to me. We were all very close and spent many weekends, holidays, and birthdays together. Almost all of our family gatherings involved a potluck where everyone brought a delicious food dish to be shared. We would then congregate in the kitchen to talk, laugh, and visit over a meal. The Filipino way is to make sure there is always more than enough food, so no one goes home hungry. We are a family that loves to bond and eat. To me food and family go hand in hand, and that continues to be a big part of my life today.

Growing up I ate mainly Filipino cuisine, consisting of a lot of starches, rice, and proteins (mostly beige food). I do vividly recall at some point when convenience food started to enter our home and meals from scratch lessened and frozen, boxed, canned, and microwave food became a go-to for my mom. I wasn't really involved in preparing or cooking meals growing up, so as I got older I also developed the habit of eating pre-prepared food. For a long time, I ate whatever was available to me without any thought.

I don't recall ever making the connection between what I ate and my health. The only time I was mindful in my food choices was if I was feeling unhappy with my body and would then diet—which consisted of eating less, rather than eating healthier. At the time, I developed the habit of associating food with body image, which sadly I think many women can relate to.

On the journey to understanding more about food and how it relates to my own health, I began educating myself to make better choices, one of which was becoming a vegetarian. In the beginning, I wasn't a healthy vegetarian. I ate a lot of processed wheat, pastas, and bread, all that really changed was that I had removed meat from my diet. Many years later, with more ups and downs, a lot of trial and error, and a whole lot more education and self-awareness, I understand more about eating the right kinds of nutrient-dense food. I know that strict diets and limiting myself doesn't work for me. I only end up quitting and going back to my old habits. I now eat a plant-based diet and being healthy has become my lifestyle, with my only goal "to feel good from the inside out."

There have been a few milestones that have prompted change. Being pregnant twice and birthing babies has given me a newfound respect for my body, what it's capable of, and how resilient it is. As a parent, I have also become responsible for the health and well-being of my children, and it's a huge responsibility—and one I don't take lightly. Having a daughter has made me realize the pressure that we as women, myself included, put on ourselves and the beauty standards we hold ourselves up against. I am slowly learning to accept, love, and appreciate myself while I redefine my idea of beauty and eat like I love myself.

Also, many years ago I completed a cleanse for the first time, and I was blown away by the results, as it completely changed the way I look at food. Over the course of a month, I had to cut out all sugar, including fruit, all dairy, all alcohol, all meat, most grains, and I ate mostly raw, plant-based foods. Without any exercise, and only following the cleanse, I had become stronger and more energetic. Along with glowing skin, I was also able to taste my food more and completely stopped craving bad food. A cleanse is intended to give your body a break and an opportunity to purify itself and, although I don't believe in restricted diets, I do periodically give my body breaks from sugar, grain, caffeine, and alcohol to reset my system.

I have been a yoga teacher for the last four years; I knew I wanted and needed to do something that I was passionate about and that would positively impact my life and others. Being in the health and wellness industry is never boring. I get to exercise my creativity, and it gives me the flexibility to maintain a healthy work/life balance.

I have the opportunity to create and run specially designed yoga programs for pregnancy, postpartum, and fertility. You can imagine how important lifestyle and nutrition are for these women. I am thrilled to involve my kids by bringing yoga into their schools and running kids' yoga camps. I am also proud to teach lunchtime classes for a department of the government as part of their wellness initiatives. More and more, I am witnessing people, communities, and organizations acknowledging the importance of a healthy lifestyle and how yoga can play a significant role in that. It is incredibly rewarding to be part of this trend.

On a personal level, since practicing yoga, I have developed a stronger self-awareness and can feel when my body isn't running optimally. My body isn't as forgiving as it was when I was younger, my metabolism has slowed down significantly, and my hormones and energy level are good indicators for when I need to clean up my diet or if I'm lacking nutrients. I need all the energy I can get as I try to keep up with the demands of a growing family.

At home, I am very aware that every moment I am teaching my kids and shaping their future as they observe me. My kids are like most, picky eaters, so whatever I make needs to taste good. They are hungry all day long and snack most of the day. Having healthy, fresh snacks readily available makes my day easier. I spend one day at the beginning of the week preparing food, washing and cutting fruits and veggies, assembling salads, making hummus, kefir, milk, and also doing some baking. It is a full day of work, but the rest of the week I don't have to think about it.

At work, I am in a position of influence, and it's important that I am leading by example. As a yoga teacher, I take a holistic and therapeutic approach in my classes, and yoga itself is intended to bridge all aspects of ourselves—body, mind, and spirit—together to make us whole. It is vital that I teach from my own experience and therefore it makes the services that I offer relevant and valuable.

LOVING HEALTHY LIVING

First and foremost, living my best health needs to feel like I'm living and not limiting or depriving myself. I have managed to make my healthy lifestyle reflect the passionate, adventurous person that I am. I know I need variety, I need food that tastes good, and I like to try new foods, new recipes, and new ingredients to keep things exciting.

Lifestyle includes my family, so we eat dinner together around the table every evening. A few years ago, I began involving my kids in gardening to get them more curious about food and, honestly, to get them to eat more vegetables, and now they look forward to planting, watering, and harvesting the garden every summer.

Another big step was cleaning out my pantry of canned and boxed foods, all wheat and white sugar, and then stocking it with some staples in our diets like quinoa, oats, nuts, dates, chia, flax, and coconut everything (oil, flakes, water, milk, sugar). I always try to load my fridge full of leafy greens, sprouts, fruits, veggies, nut butters, and milk.

Last, but most important, is prioritizing myself. I am now able to see that cooking and eating are self-care practices. Taking the time to cook and eat what I enjoy, and not just what my family wants, is practicing self-care. It is also acknowledging when I need a break and deciding to go out for a meal or pick something up instead. Along with self-care comes self-love, and I no longer focus on body image, I honor my body by listening to what it needs, and I really just try to implement balance in my life.

Drinking lots of water has definitely had the most impact on my health. Growing up I drank juice and pop, and today, aside from a cup of coffee in the morning and herbal tea in the evening, I drink water all day long, and it helps to keep me feeling young and energetic.

About ten years ago I was introduced to drinking and making my own kefir, a probiotic drink, and have since continued to make a smoothie for my family every morning. It's had a life-changing effect on my gut health, I rarely get sick with colds or the flu, and I would definitely attribute that to the kefir.

Of course, the decision to eat a plant-based diet not only feels good ethically, but it has also drastically improved my energy level and digestion. Eating nutrient-dense food truly does impact our health physically, energetically, emotionally, and mentally. That's a big deal.

Cooking nutrient-dense food can taste amazing and be easy to prepare. Balance is key! Eat what you want to, but do it in moderation and/or find a healthier version of it. I love chocolate and have found a way to eat it without any guilt (recipe on following pages).

It is important to get inspired about food, eating, and cooking.

Here are some things that help to inspire me:

- Splurge on a gorgeous cookbook and try everything in it. I love *Oh She Glows* and *Whitewater Cooks*, both from Canadian authors.

- Follow some awesome food bloggers on Instagram and see daily pictures of their beautiful recipes and often quick, easy-to-follow videos. I love Minimalist Baker (@minimalistbaker) and Erin Ireland (@erinireland).

- My go-to for inspiration, hands down, is Pinterest. Set up an account, then search and save all kinds of recipes in one place. Disclaimer: You may become addicted.

- As a family, we love watching cooking shows, and our favorite is Master Chef.

- Host a potluck for friends; that way, everyone shares in the cooking, and you can try new dishes plus swap recipes. Bonus: You can bond over food and wine and share in the clean-up.

We are all different, and what works for me may not be what works for you, so get in your kitchen and experiment. Try new recipes and new ingredients. Play aroud with making your food look pretty, and you'll enjoy eating it that much more.

Eat like you love yourself and remember to put yourself and your well-being first!

> "Be the change you wish to see in the world."
>
> **Mahatma Gandhi**

Nicole Jennifer Enns

Yoga Instructor
Chilliwack, British Columbia

RAW ENERGY BALLS

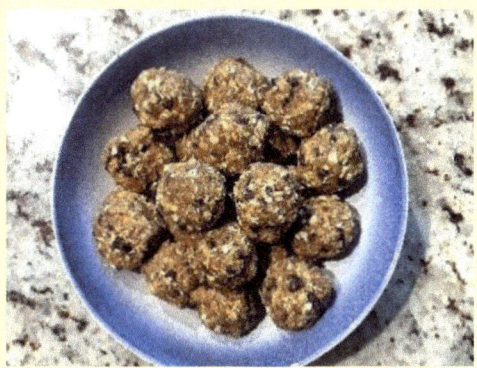

Calories	203
Protein	5g
CHO	21g
Fat	11g
Sugar	14g
Sodium	50mg
Fiber	3g
Chol	0mg

Makes up to 25 balls, keeps in the fridge for about 7 days.

Per energy ball

INGREDIENTS

- ½ cup pumpkin seeds
- ½ cup dry rolled oats (I use gluten-free.)
- ½ cup toasted shredded coconut
- ½ cup flax meal
- ½ cup peanut butter or almond butter
- ½ cup mini chocolate chips (I use vegan.)
- ⅓ cup honey or maple syrup
- 1 teaspoon vanilla extract

Optional

- Dried fruit, chia seeds, hemp seeds

DIRECTIONS

Thoroughly mix all ingredients together in a bowl. Cover and place in the fridge to chill approximately 30 minutes.

Once chilled, hand roll into bite-sized balls and store in a sealed container. If mixture is too wet, add more oats. If mixture is too dry, add more nut butter.

COCONUT OIL CHOCOLATE SQUARES

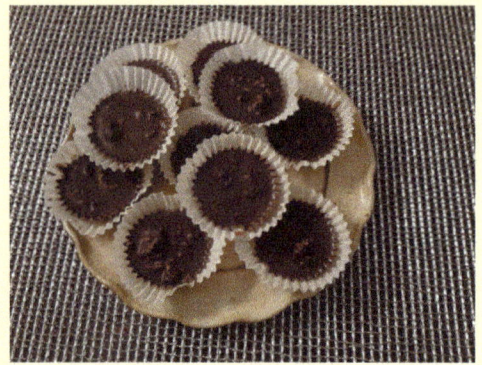

Calories	49
Protein	0g
CHO	1g
Fat	4g
Sugar	0g
Sodium	5mg
Fiber	1g
Chol	0mg

Makes 32 squares

Per square

INGREDIENTS

- 2 ice cube trays or small muffin tin
- ½ cup cold pressed unrefined coconut oil
- ½ cup cacao (cocoa also works)
- pinch Himalayan salt
- 1 to 2 tablespoons sweetener, coconut sugar, maple syrup, or honey
- Chef's Note: Xylitol can be used as a sweetener for diabetic option (be sure to keep away from pets).

Extras

- chopped nuts, seeds, dried fruit, flaked coconut, peanut butter
- You can also experiment with flavor extracts like vanilla, peppermint, and orange, but use sparingly.

DIRECTIONS

Prepare the ice cube trays by filling the bottom quarter of each tray with your nuts or whichever extra ingredients you have chosen. (I enjoy variety and generally make 4 different kinds, which would give me 6 squares of each.)

Add the coconut oil, cacao, salt, extract, and sweetener to a saucepan and stir on low heat until completed melted and mixed together. (If using honey as sweetener, wait until the chocolate mixture cools before adding the honey so you don't kill its natural enzymes.)

Pour a spoonful of the melted chocolate mixture into each ice cube square and place into the freezer until solid, about 1 to 2 hours.

Once firm, they can be kept in a sealed container in the refrigerator for up to 2 weeks, but you know you'll eat them all long before that.

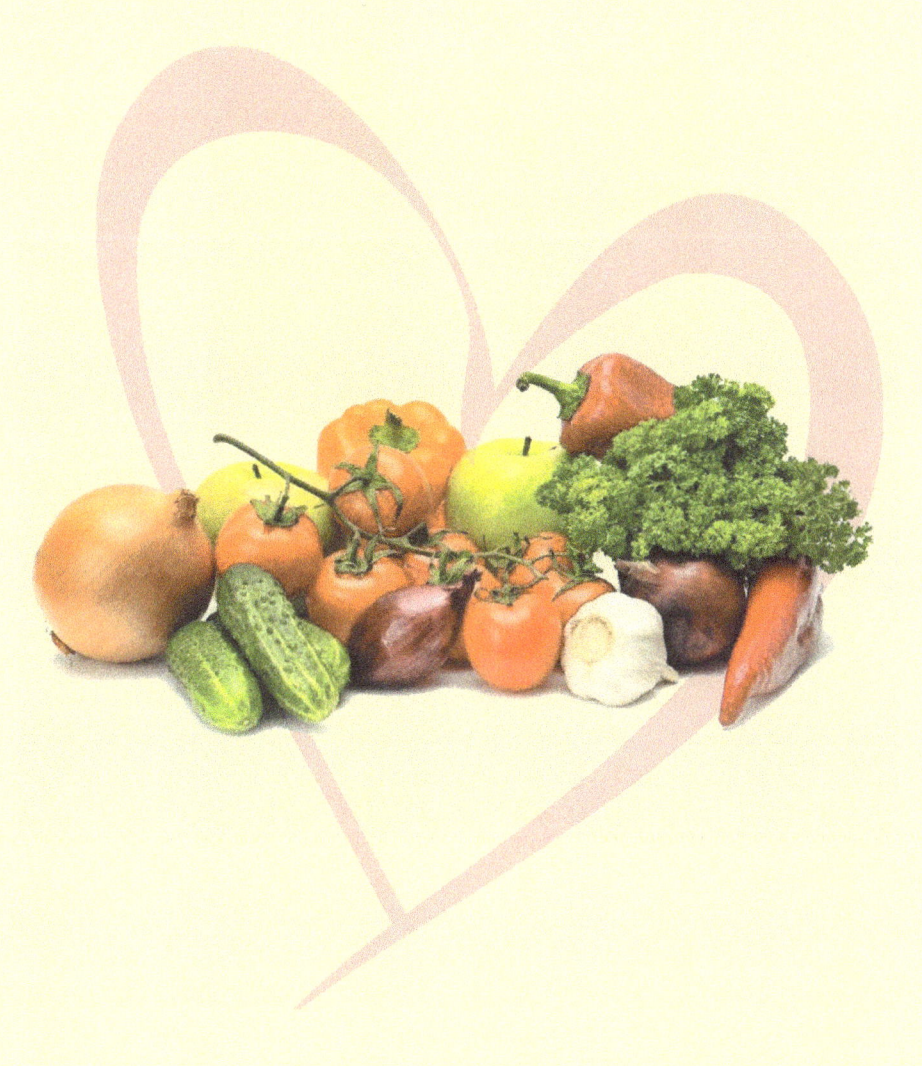

CHANGE THE WORLD ONE PLATE AT A TIME

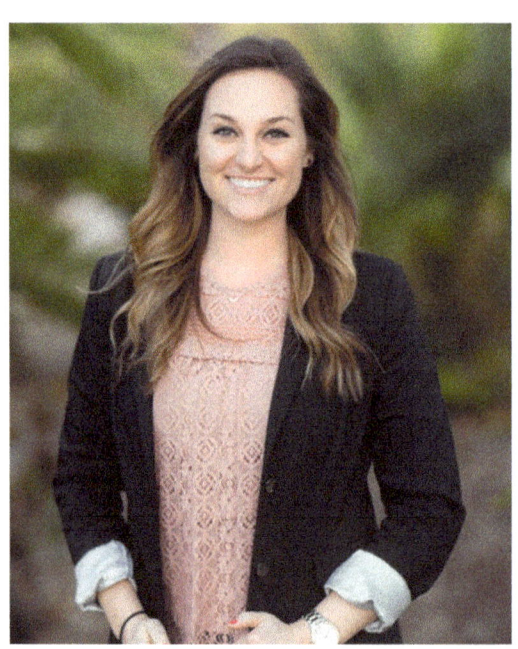

Brittany Johnson

I grew up in a loving, Christian home in Beaumont, California. Life growing up was always an adventure. I was an active kid, constantly outside playing. However, I struggled with an eating disorder while growing up, restricting my calories to be thin. On top of that, I was a very picky eater and didn't have much variety in my diet. After taking a nutrition class in college, I fell in love with the science. Understanding the concept of food as fuel allowed me to develop a healthier relationship with food.

Food is a powerful tool that can heal or damage our bodies. Each day we have an opportunity to optimize our health by what we eat. I now have the honor of teaching college students and athletes about my passion for nutrition and health. Seeing people transform themselves through healthful eating and lifestyle changes gives me a great sense of satisfaction. I love to help spread the healthy eating message through educating students about the science-based evidence. Teaching in higher education affords me opportunities to research and teach my passion. Most of all, I love seeing people change their lives through nutrition education.

One step I have taken to better my health is simply making it a priority. I wake up early to spend time with God in devotion, eat a light breakfast, then head off to the gym. Setting aside time for yourself is essential. We need to celebrate everything our bodies do for us daily. If there is any advice I would share, it is to take it slowly and give yourself grace. We can't radically change everything about our diet and lifestyle overnight. Small changes create a ripple effect. Cheers to health!

> Change the world one plate at a time.

Brittany Johnson

MS, RDN, CSSD
Assistant Professor of Nutrition, Dietetics and Food
Point Loma Nazarene University
Certified Specialist of Sports Dietetics
brittanyjohnson@pointloma.edu

HEALTHY SPICED BANANA BREAD

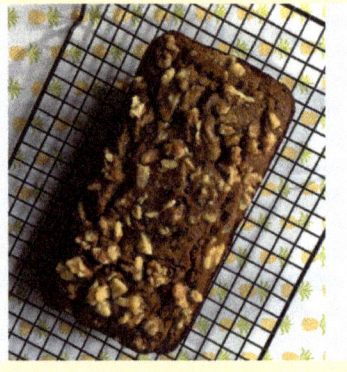

Calories	224
Protein	4g
CHO	34g
Fat	8g
Sugar	19g
Sodium	308mg
Fiber	4g
Chol	0mg

Makes 1 loaf

Per slice

INGREDIENTS

- 3 ripe bananas
- 2 egg whites
- ¼ cup canola oil
- ¼ cup applesauce
- ¾ cup sugar
- 1 cup whole wheat flour
- ¾ cup all-purpose flour
- 1 teaspoon baking soda
- ¾ teaspoon salt
- 1 teaspoon cinnamon
- 1 teaspoon nutmeg
- ¼ cup chopped walnuts (optional)

Nothing compares the aroma of freshly baked banana bread. A go-to morning snack usually includes coffee and a pastry. Blending my love of baking and passion for nutrition, I'm on a pursuit to improve the nutritional quality of high-fat, high-sugar goodies. That's exactly what this recipe does!

DIRECTIONS

Preheat oven to 350°F. Mix the wet ingredients—bananas, egg whites, canola oil, and applesauce—in a large bowl and set aside.

Mix dry ingredients—sugar, whole wheat flour, all-purpose flour, baking soda, salt, cinnamon, nutmeg—in a medium bowl. Fold dry ingredients into wet ingredients until just moistened.

Top with chopped nuts, if desired, and bake for 50–55 minutes.

VEGGIE EGG WHITE MUFFINS

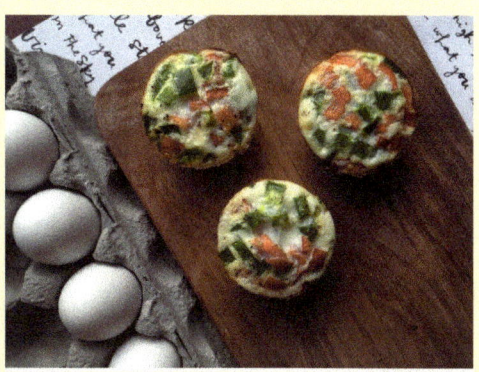

Calories	24
Protein	4g
CHO	1g
Fat	0g
Sugar	0g
Sodium	75mg
Fiber	0g
Chol	0mg

Makes 12 muffins

Per 1 muffin

INGREDIENTS

- nonstick cooking spray
- 1 quart real liquid egg whites
- ¼ cup chopped green pepper
- ¼ cup chopped red pepper
- ¼ cup chopped green onions
- ¼ cup diced fresh tomatoes
- pinch of black pepper
- pinch of garlic powder

DIRECTIONS

- Spray 12 muffins tins with nonstick spray.
- Fill muffin tins halfway with chopped veggies.
- Pour real liquid egg whites to the top.
- Sprinkle pepper and garlic powder.
- Bake for 25 minutes at 350ºF.

LET FOOD BE THY MEDICINE

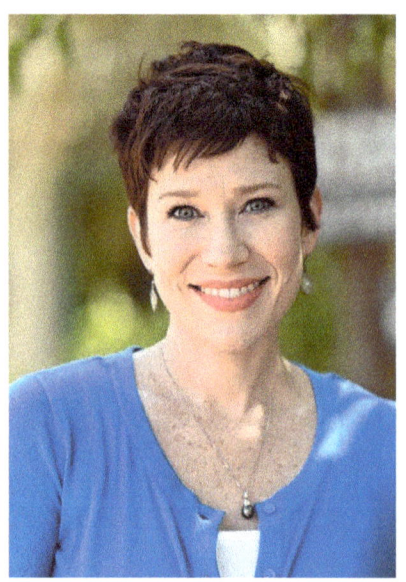

Hollie Ancharoff

I grew up in a small town in southeastern Kentucky. Beautiful country, rolling hills, and enormous backyard gardens characterized my childhood. I clearly remember working in the garden in the summertime, as well knowing it would be "all hands on deck" when harvest time came. Preserving the summer's bounty the old-fashioned way through canning, drying, and freezing meant that everyone had to work together. If you dropped into my grandmother's house anytime from late summer through fall, you'd quickly be given a job stringing or breaking beans, shucking corn, peeling apples, canning tomatoes, or making berry preserves. There was such beauty growing up in a place where there was a tradition of growing and preserving your own food, and the benefits were more than simply filling next year's pantry. Many of my favorite childhood memories include being taught the right way to plant tomatoes, watching the squash blossoms turn into vegetables, and breaking beans with my great-grandmother—a silver paring knife and a bowl of beans were a permanent fixture on her lap in the summer. She did the stringing, and my young fingers did the breaking.

Yet, as I grew older, one unfortunate consequence of being located directly on busy Interstate 75 was the sprouting up of a multitude of fast food restaurants. My small home town once claimed four McDonald's! As life got busier with two working parents and many after school activities, eating this kind of food became the norm. We still had Sunday dinners at grandmas, but often the preserved vegetables were accompanied by an easy-to-add bucket of Kentucky Fried Chicken— that chain was even born in my hometown. You could visit the original Sander's Café and Museum and "Eat Where it all Began."

The damage from eating lots of fried fast food, starchy French fries and soda, and low-quality, hormone-laden meats could not be undone by a moderate amount of fresh vegetables. Soon I began to suffer from debilitating endometriosis and ovarian cysts, as well as cystic acne and frequent allergies and sinus infections. These symptoms led to a host of medical interventions; over my teenage and college years, I was prescribed frequent rounds of antibiotics, a range of hormone therapies, surgery for endometriosis, sinus surgery and tonsillectomy, as well as various medications for allergies and asthma. At one point, at only twenty-two years of age, I counted my ongoing prescriptions: nine! Intuitively I knew there had to be a better solution.

My first experiment in taking charge of my own health was to try going vegetarian—my mother was also an endometriosis sufferer and had read that the hormones in meat and dairy, as well as plastic components such as BPA and dioxins, could influence endometriosis. I eliminated cooking, microwaving, and drinking water from plastic, switched to organic dairy, and stopped eating meat. The endometriosis disappeared quickly, never to return, but my journey was far from over. Over the next several years, I still struggled with acne, allergies, low energy, and a brush with gestational diabetes. The gestational diabetes regimen increased my awareness of just how laden my diet was with inflammatory carbs. I relied heavily on wheat, pasta, and gluten-based meat substitutes. Eventually I stumbled across the work of Dr. Loren Cordain, researcher and creator of the paleo diet. I discovered that my acne was likely caused by a combination of gluten, dairy, and sugar. I did add meats back to my diet in small amounts but insisted that they be high quality, hormone free and humanely raised. My energy increased and my allergies disappeared, but my acne lingered.

One day I picked up *The Virgin Diet* by J.J. Virgin and discovered that many people have sensitivity to eggs. I was dubious, but since dietary changes had always solved my symptoms before, I gave it a try. After just two weeks egg-free, my acne finally completely disappeared!

What does my diet look like now? I call it a plant-based paleo template. I eat a small amount of very high-quality meat and fish, lots of healthy fats such as nuts, seeds, grass-fed butter, olive and avocado oils, a sprinkling of low-sugar fruit and low-glycemic starchy vegetables such as sweet potatoes and carrots, and lots of non-starchy green vegetables. While not everyone is completely intolerant of grains, legumes, dairy, sugar, eggs, or gluten, my sensitivity to so many foods likely resulted from the years of antibiotics disrupting my gut microbiome. It's also likely that I always had a mild dairy/gluten intolerance that was worsened when those foods comprised much of my diet. The focus now is on gut friendly, low glycemic, high nutrient, healing foods.

I decided to become a health coach because it took me years to navigate the confusing and conflicting avalanche of information about which "diet" is best. If I'd had a guide to help me try an elimination diet early on, I could have saved myself years of suffering, expense, and medical intervention. The energy and health I experience as a result of eliminating food sensitivities is profound. The message I'd most like to communicate to people is that if you are suffering from health problems or low energy, you are not crazy! As Hippocrates said, "Let food be thy medicine." Use your body as an experimentation lab to eliminate and then reintroduce foods that commonly cause sensitivity. Don't be afraid to test everything! While it might seem daunting, getting to the root of which foods work best for your body is not limiting—it is liberating. There is nothing more empowering than focusing on a diet that makes you feel incredible!

> ... and as we let our own light shine, we subconsciously give others permission to do the same. As we are liberated from our fear our presence automatically liberates others. So it's holy work—to move past your own fear. It doesn't just help you, it helps the world.

Marianne Williamson

Hollie Ancharoff

Certified Health Coach
Long Beach, California
Email: hollieancharoff@gmail.com
www.hollieancharoff.com

FENNEL AND ORANGE SALAD

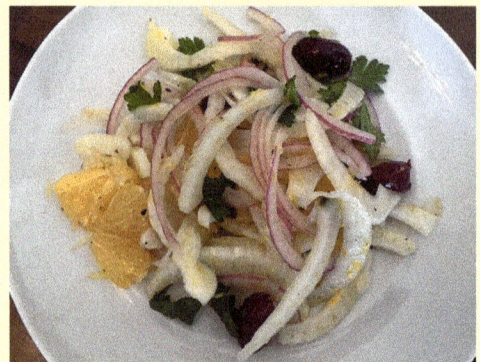

Calories	235
Protein	2g
CHO	23g
Fat	15g
Sugar	13g
Sodium	238mg
Fiber	8g
Chol	0mg

Serves 4

Per serving

This salad is really a traditional Italian dish I learned from my sister. I like to add onion to the salad, as well as fresh orange juice, zest, and vinegar to the dressing for a little more kick than the simplest traditional version. The salad makes great use of fennel, which I believe to be a very underappreciated vegetable! It also holds up well without wilting when dressed, so it makes a great dish for gatherings or for leftovers.

INGREDIENTS

For the salad

- 2 large fennel bulbs
- 2 medium oranges (1 for juicing)
- ½ medium red onion, sliced
- ¼ cup pitted Kalamata olives
- handful of Italian parsley

For the dressing

- ½ cup olive oil
- ¼ cup white wine or tarragon vinegar
- 2 tablespoons freshly squeezed orange juice
- 2 teaspoons orange zest
- pinch of salt, to taste
- freshly ground black pepper, to taste

DIRECTIONS

Zest one of the oranges and juice half, then place the resulting juice and zest in a small bowl. Using a sharp knife remove the peel and pith from the remaining oranges. First, cut the oranges into ¼-inch-round slices, then cut in half again to make half-moon shapes and add to a mixing bowl. Slice the red onion the same way and add to the bowl. Trim a few of the green fennel fronds for garnish, then slice the fennel bulbs down the middle and remove the tough core. Using either a very sharp knife or a mandolin, slice the fennel into thin half-moons and add to the bowl. Roughly tear or chop the parsley and add.

Add all dressing ingredients to the small bowl and whisk, then pour over the salad, add Kalamata olives, then toss. Taste for seasoning and add more salt and pepper if desired. Pour salad onto serving plate or bowl and sprinkle with fennel fronds.

COCONUT, BERRY & PECAN CEREAL

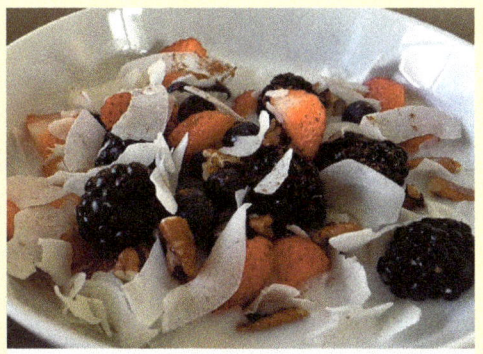

Calories	335
Protein	6g
CHO	21g
Fat	28g
Sugar	11g
Sodium	145mg
Fiber	8g
Chol	0mg

Serves 2

Per serving

Although this is quite a simple "recipe," it's brimming with healthful ingredients, is low in sugar, and satisfies a real craving for folks who need to avoid grains but miss the feeling of having a bowl of breakfast cereal. The nuts and coconut shavings add cereal-like crunch, and the berries taste wonderful with a creamy dairy-milk alternative. It's one of my favorite additions to my diet.

INGREDIENTS

- 1 cup any organic berries
- ½ cup unsweetened coconut chips/shavings
- ¼ cup pecans (my favorite, walnuts are great too!) roughly broken or chopped
- 1 cup almond milk, or any dairy milk alternative
- tiny pinch of salt
- sprinkle of any warming spice such as nutmeg, cinnamon, or cardamom.

DIRECTIONS

Add all ingredients to a bowl and enjoy!

Here are several options for changing it up:

- Change the kind of berries or nuts.
- Experiment with adding seeds such as ground flax, chia, sunflower, or pepitas.
- Try different sprinklings of spice or a drizzle of honey.
- Try roasting the nuts or seeds.
- Try warming the milk, berries, and chia seeds gently in a saucepan, then stir in coconut and nuts for a delicious grain-free "hot cereal" alternative.

I GOT MY LIFE BACK

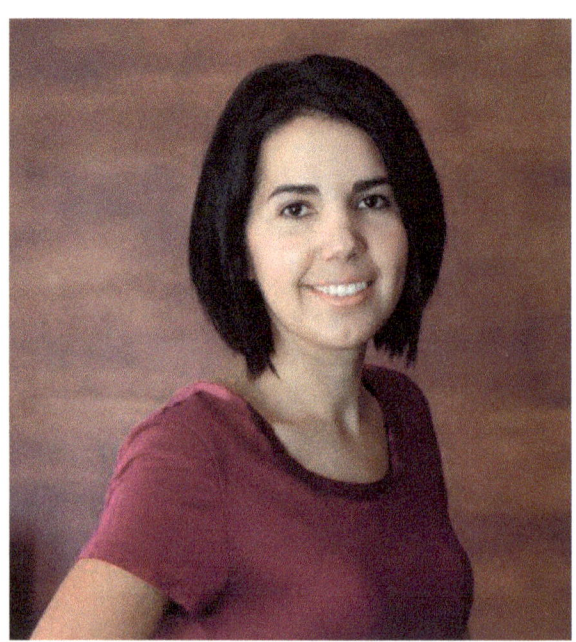

Amber Anderson

I grew up in Salt Lake City, Utah, and as a child I had no interest in healthy food. Like most kids, it was all about the sweets for me. I did eat other foods besides sweets; however, my diet wasn't very balanced despite my parents trying to have me eat vegetables with most meals. As I grew up, my taste buds did change. I started to eat healthier; however, that doesn't mean I gave up my sweet tooth. At the age of nineteen, I noticed I was growing increasingly tired and that my friends had more energy and ambition than I did. I began to feel like something was wrong with me, that I must be lazy or that I had a personality flaw. At this time, I also started to develop allergies, and I thought it was a result of the environment, such as dust, dander, plants, and the general air quality where I lived.

Through my twenties, my symptoms became increasingly worse, and to say I was tired was an understatement. Most days I would take a nap, yet I would still go to bed early and sleep ten to eleven hours. I had hoped that after that much sleep, I would at least wake up refreshed, but I didn't and wasn't sure if this was normal or not. As a young mother at the age of twenty-three with small children, it seemed like that was the reason I was feeling so drained. Then when I turned thirty, my health took a real downward spiral. I was thirty-five pounds heavier than I had ever been, and exercise wasn't working for me like it had in the past. I started to get a rash on my face that looked like I was going through puberty. Plus, I noticed that I was slowly becoming more irritable and at times this problem was in overdrive. I snapped at everyone I loved, constantly seemed depressed, and didn't enjoy the things that I really loved and wanted most in my life. I was never great at multi-tasking, but at this time I couldn't even think clearly—on top of this, I was becoming more forgetful. I would get overwhelmed and withdraw from others, which took a big toll on my family, especially my children. It was a very difficult time, as I was a different person than I wanted to be.

During this difficult time, I had a very nice neighbor give me some advice. She suggested I try going off gluten and see if that would help me. I wasn't really open to the idea of getting rid of a food that I loved so much. I couldn't imagine what I would eat instead. So I ignored her advice. Four years later, all those symptoms had increased significantly. It was an emotional time for me, as I cried on the floor of my bedroom, thinking I was too young to be feeling this sick. I knew something had to change.

Then I discovered something amazing—my neighbor was right! Initially, the learning came as a result of looking for some way to help my children with their struggles at school. In my research, I learned that going off gluten can help kids with learning challenges (which my kids were dealing with). As a mother, I would do anything for my children, so as a family we went off gluten for two weeks to see if we noticed any differences. I had no intention of going off gluten completely for myself, but if it helped my kids, I was willing to do it for them. It was the best gift of my life when my children and I began to feel better, happier, and experience more energy. We decided there was no going back to eating gluten. My "allergies" went away, my skin cleared up, exercise became affective again, and I could think more clearly than ever before.

Unfortunately for me, I had waited a little too long to discover the beauty of going gluten-free. Because I was on gluten so long, I developed an autoimmune disease called Hashimoto's thyroiditis. I have found a wonderful doctor who is helping me heal and, in the meantime, I inform people who are just not feeling quite themselves that they can help heal their bodies through the foods they eat. Sickness can be prevented simply by make some diet changes. You don't have to live life feeling sluggish and drained. Now, I feel more alive and have more energy in my mid-thirties than I did in my twenties. I understand that I don't have a personality flaw, and I'm discovering what I am truly made of. I became a health coach so I could help others, who are having challenges with their health, to overcome their symptoms and to help them live the life they only dream of.

Eliminating gluten can seem daunting and time consuming, but imagine if you have more energy as a result. Energy creates so many opportunities in life and allows us to engage in the beauty of living. Once you have more energy to live, you will be able to focus more on eating foods that give you energy, and you will move away from foods that take your energy away. Learning what foods your body needs is the first step to healthy, vibrant living. Having energy is like having more time to take better care of yourself, so you can give your best self to the ones you love.

> *Only when it is dark enough can you see the stars.*
>
> **Martin Luther King Jr.**

Amber Anderson

Certified Health Coach
Farmington, Utah
www.habitrebel.com

KID-APPROVED ALLERGY-FRIENDLY PUMPKIN MUFFINS

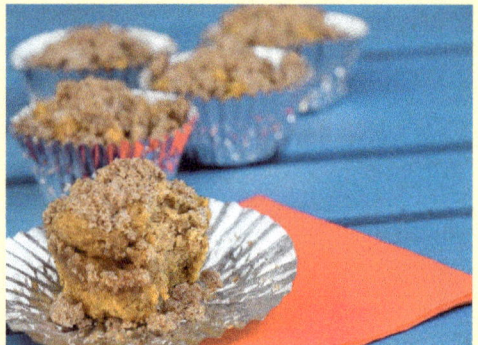

Calories	200
Protein	3g
CHO	22g
Fat	13g
Sugar	19g
Sodium	71mg
Fiber	2g
Chol	0mg

Makes 10 muffins

Per muffin

INGREDIENTS

- 1 ½ cups gluten-free almond flour
- 1 teaspoon guar gum (if guar gum or xanthan gum isn't already included in the flour)
- 2 teaspoons baking powder
- ¼ teaspoon salt
- 1 ½ teaspoons cinnamon
- ½ teaspoon nutmeg
- ¼ teaspoon ground cloves
- 2 tablespoons ground flax seeds

- 6 tablespoons warm water
- ½ cup almond milk
- ¼ cup pure maple syrup
- 3 tablespoons olive oil
- 1 teaspoon pure vanilla
- ½ cup pureed pumpkin
- ½ teaspoon black pepper
- ¼ teaspoon curry powder
- ⅛ teaspoon garlic powder
- ⅛ teaspoon cinnamon

DIRECTIONS

Preheat oven to 350°F. Line muffin tin with baking cups.

Mix ground flaxseed with warm water, set aside. In a large bowl mix gluten-free flour, guar gum, baking powder, salt, cinnamon, nutmeg, clove, then set aside. In a small saucepan, whisk together almond milk, maple syrup, olive oil, vanilla, and pureed pumpkin until melted together.

Add liquid mixture and soaking ground flax seeds to dry ingredients. Stir until fully mixed.

Add batter to baking cups. Muffins won't rise much, so fill the cups to the top. Add crumble (recipe next page) to the top of the muffin batter.

Bake 20 minutes or until toothpick comes out clean. Move muffins to cooling rack to cool. Muffin texture is best when it is completely cool.

CRUMBLE TOPPING

- ¾ cup gluten-free almond flour
- ½ cup coconut palm sugar
- ½ teaspoon cinnamon
- ¼ teaspoon nutmeg
- ¼ teaspoon clove
- 4 tablespoons unrefined olive oil

Make crumble by mixing flour, coconut palm sugar, cinnamon, nutmeg, clove, and olive oil; set aside. Crumble will top 20 muffins.

KID APPROVED ALLERGY FREE WAFFLES

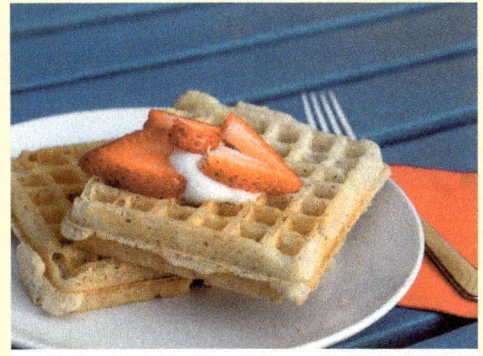

	Per serving
Calories	191
Protein	2g
CHO	28g
Fat	9g
Sugar	1g
Sodium	347mg
Fiber	2g
Chol	0mg

Makes about 8 servings

INGREDIENTS

- 2 tablespoons ground flax seeds
- 1 cup brown rice flour
- ½ cup potato starch*
- ¼ cup tapioca flour
- 2 teaspoons baking powder
- 1 teaspoon salt
- ¼ cup olive oil
- 6 tablespoons warm water
- 1 ½ cups unsweetened nut milk
- 1 teaspoon raw agave syrup

DIRECTIONS

Mix ground flax seed with warm water, set aside for 10 minutes. Mix all ingredients together, including soaking ground flax seed, with beater. Batter will be thick. If you prefer a thinner batter, add a bit more milk. Put about ⅓ cup batter in for each waffle. Cook in a waffle iron about 3–4 minutes depending on how crispy you like your waffles. Top with any topping you like.

*Not potato flour

A JOURNEY TO BETTER HEALTH

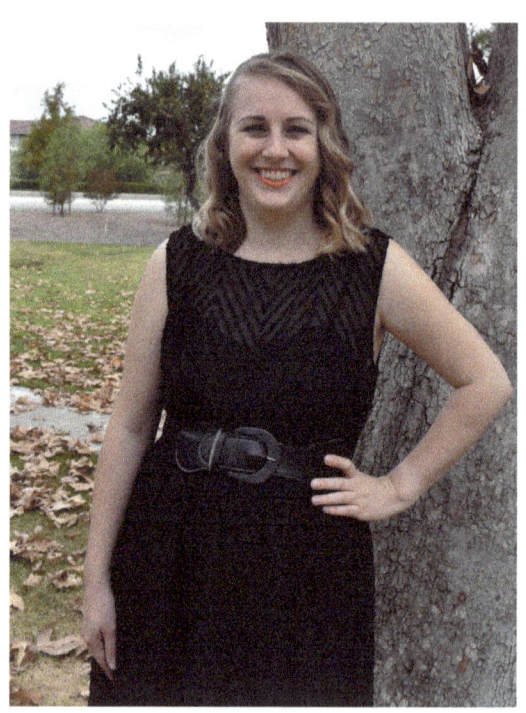

Kirsten Ault

I grew up in a small town in California where my parents owned two acres of land and had a garden with a variety of fruits and vegetables right at their fingertips. The garden included tomatoes, corn, asparagus, potatoes, cabbage, carrots, beets, onions, garlic, squash, broccoli, oranges, peaches, plums, watermelon, cherries, cantaloupe, and apricots. It was like having our own personal grocery store. This sparked my initial interest in food and continued to grow as I watched the process of planting, picking, and cooking the food we grew.

My childhood was an active one where I was in dance classes three to four days a week from the ages of three to fifteen. We would have home cooked meals as a family most nights of the week. As a child, I would eat most foods except for Brussels sprouts and fish, from what I remember. I would watch my mom cook in the kitchen and help her sometimes, but most of the time the kitchen scared me (I am not really sure why). Nowadays, my eating habits haven't changed too much, except for loving Brussels sprouts and fish, and roasted vegetables have been one of my favorite things to make as a side for dinner. I love experimenting with different spices and recipes; it's like a science experiment.

One experience that led me to nutrition began when I was in middle school. I was in the fourth grade and kept getting these unbearable headaches and could not figure out the cause; eventually I found out what foods triggered those headaches. I would write down everything I would eat throughout the day and figure out what was causing the pain. I still suffer from headaches to this day, but I can pretty much tell what causes them: not enough sleep, not eating enough throughout the day, eating a trigger food, etc. I learned that I needed to eat every two to three hours to keep my energy levels up and make sure I did not get a headache.

During high school, I was diagnosed with Gastroparesis after many visits to doctors and various specialists. I had a test called the Gastric Emptying Test, where I was required to eat food prior to the test and have a camera hanging over my stomach for one hour to see how fast the food passed through my GI tract. The result was telling. After one hour, the food I consumed had not moved very far in the digesting stage in my stomach. I had to change my diet with this diagnosis, starting with liquids, and slowly advancing my diet to help with the pain. After a few months, I had no issue with it; the doctors believed it was from a virus.

One of the main reasons I chose nutrition was my grandparents' diet and lifestyle habits catching up with them. My grandma was diagnosed as a Type II diabetic, and her disease gradually continued to worsen. Six years later, her kidney function decreased, and she was put on dialysis immediately.

My grandpa was a smoker all his life and ate whatever he wanted. Eventually he was diagnosed as a Type II diabetic and later diagnosed with stage 4 lung cancer. Watching them have to check blood sugars, give insulin, take medications, be on dialysis, and go through chemotherapy—and see them go through so much pain and agony—was heartbreaking. This was a turning point in my life; I knew I wanted to pursue a career in nutrition. Sadly, both of them have passed, and I was devastated. But I made a promise to myself that I would make them proud by becoming a Registered Dietitian. I strive to live a healthier lifestyle for my grandparents and family with easy tips such as shopping around the perimeter of the store where the produce, meats, dairy are located, cooking meals using spices other than salt and pepper, and exercising at least thirty minutes every day.

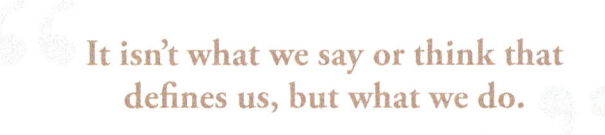

It isn't what we say or think that defines us, but what we do.

Jane Austen

Kirsten Ault, RDN

Menifee, California
Email: ault.kirstenj@gmail.com

BLACK BEAN AND ZUCCHINI TACOS

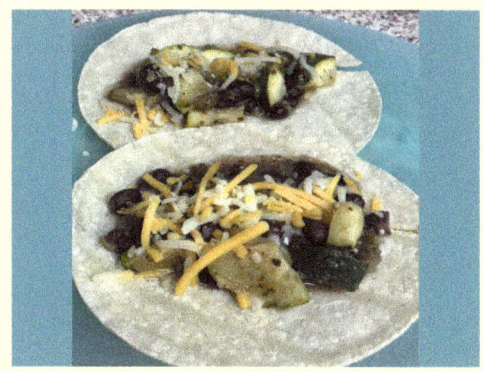

Calories	136
Protein	5g
CHO	23g
Fat	3g
Sugar	3g
Sodium	160mg
Fiber	6g
Chol	0mg

Serves 8

Per taco

INGREDIENTS

- 2 medium zucchini, cut into rounds, then quartered
- 2 cups homemade black beans (recipe next page)
- 1 tablespoon olive oil
- 1 cup salsa verde
- 8 homemade corn tortillas (see recipe next page)

DIRECTIONS

Cut zucchini into rounds and cut into quarters.

Cook black beans (recipe next page) in slow cooker the night before.

Heat pan with 1 tablespoon of olive oil.

Add zucchini and cook until lightly browned, approximately 6–8 minutes.

Add black beans to zucchini, cook for 1–2 minutes.

Add salsa verde to zucchini and black beans.

Simmer for 5 minutes or until everything is hot.

Serve on homemade corn tortillas.

Feel free to add other toppings as garnishes, such as avocado, cheese (or soy cheese of choice), tomatoes, etc.

See homemade corn tortilla recipe (next page).

HOMEMADE BLACK BEANS

Makes 5 cups

INGREDIENTS

- 16 ounces dry black beans
- 1 small onion, chopped
- 1 clove garlic, chopped
- 1 tablespoon chopped fresh cilantro
- ¼ teaspoon cayenne pepper
- Salt to taste

Calories	113
Protein	7g
CHO	22g
Fat	0g
Sugar	1g
Sodium	10mg
Fiber	7g
Chol	0mg

Per ½ cup

Drain and rinse beans. Place beans, onion, garlic, cilantro, and cayenne pepper in slow cooker. Cook for 6–8 hours on low or 3–4 hours on high. Salt to taste.

HOMEMADE CORN TORTILLAS

Makes 12 tortillas

INGREDIENTS

- 1 ¾ cups masa harina
- 1 ⅛ cups water

Calories	58
Protein	1g
CHO	12g
Fat	1g
Sugar	0g
Sodium	0mg
Fiber	1g
Chol	0mg

Per tortilla

DIRECTIONS

In a medium bowl, mix together masa harina and hot water until thoroughly combined. Turn dough onto a clean surface and knead until pliable and smooth. If dough is too sticky, add more masa harina; if it begins to dry out, sprinkle with water. Cover dough tightly with plastic wrap and allow to stand for 30 minutes.

Preheat a cast iron skillet or griddle to medium-high.

Divide dough into 12 equally sized balls. Using a tortilla press, or your hands, press each ball of dough flat between two sheets of plastic wrap.

Immediately place tortilla in preheated pan and allow to cook for approximately 30 seconds, or until browned and slightly puffy. Turn tortilla over to brown on second side for approximately 30 seconds more, then transfer to a plate. Repeat process with each ball of dough. Keep tortillas covered with a towel to stay warm and moist until ready to serve.

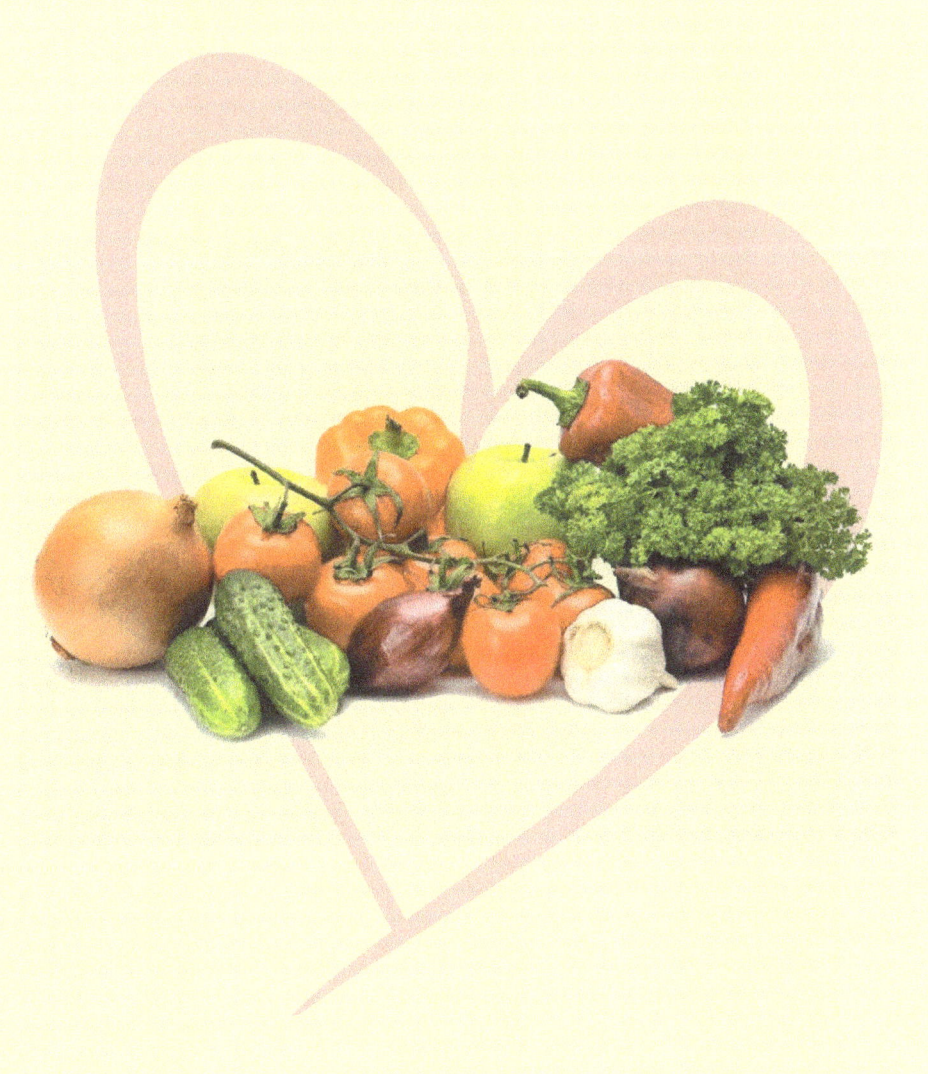

NEW HABITS BETTER LIFE

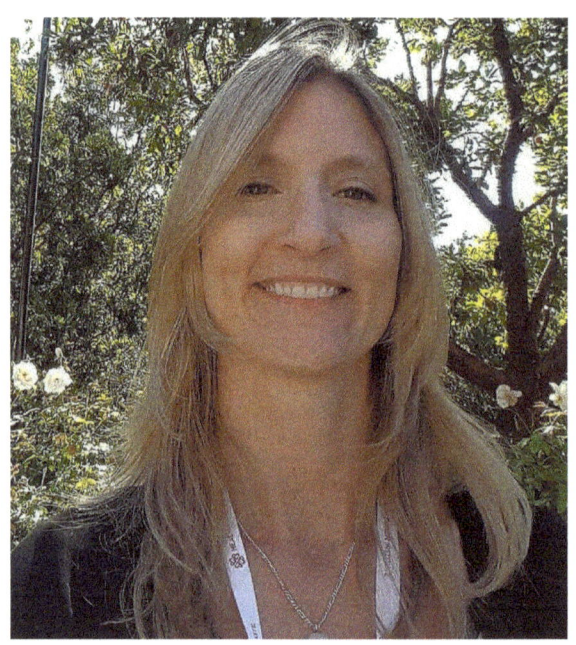

Holly Kelsey

I grew up in Westminster, Colorado, and was very close to my grandparents, who nurtured me and are responsible for my simple approach to cooking. They also helped me at an early age to begin saving for my future. My mom was also a great role model; she encouraged me in school and taught me that education was the key to my future. Tennis was my favorite sport growing up, but I also loved to play musical instruments. I enjoyed the outdoors and spent much of my time riding my bicycle, which gave me a feeling of freedom.

Growing up, my family cooked meals on more of a traditional basis, which included some type of bread at nearly every meal and, if not bread, pasta. I also recall eating a lot of tomatoes but most all of our meals included some form of carbohydrates. After school, I loved to snack on a chunk of cheese or celery with peanut butter, followed by my favorite chocolate candy bar or the most common doughnut at the time.

As an adult, I found it difficult to maintain the same amount of activity as I did as a child, which resulted in being more lethargic and having excess weight. Many days my body felt achy all over and, after some visits to a doctor, it was suggested that I may have fibromyalgia. My throat often was sore from drainage, and my breathing was impacted. In attempts to correct the sinus issue, I had two rhinoplasty surgeries but neither corrected the problem. My hair grew thin and brittle, and I was having pain in my bladder. Depression was a harsh reality at the time.

So I decided to change my eating habits to see if that would help. It was a learning process and, through the elimination of certain foods, I discovered that I had a strong negative reaction to gluten. By eliminating gluten, I was able to see my body slim down with very little effort. My energy came back, and my aches and pains went away. Best of all, my sinus issue was solved! I could breathe, swallow normally, and my throat stopped feeling scratchy and sore. My hair began growing in thicker, darker, and with more body! An ALCAT test confirmed that gluten had, indeed, caused my body inflammation at a cellular level.

So today, when I eat gluten, I suffer. All of those miserable symptoms I had start to reappear. Because wheat gluten is added to most processed foods, I have learned to be creative in the kitchen and to modify recipes to be gluten-free. I find that I now eat more vegetables, fruit, and clean proteins, organic whenever possible. I don't avoid carbohydrates, but I do try to limit them to simple carbohydrates. The energy I have gained from eating nutritiously has transformed my life. I now have more time to enjoy a variety of exercises like hiking, dancing, playing, and enjoying life more. I even get a few bike rides in now and again!

Before going out to eat, I do some research on restaurants I would like to visit and learn what their gluten-free menu is like, then I can figure out how I can edit some of their foods in order to eat gluten-free. Now that I have a better understanding of my problem and how to adjust my life accordingly, it doesn't feel so daunting. As a result of making some minor adjustments to the foods I eat, the benefits have been awesome. I no longer have to worry about future surgeries, and there is no need for medications to reduce the pain. I now am happy and feel much healthier.

Because of the things I have learned through my own health challenges, I have chosen a career to teach others how to live healthier and to reduce or eliminate their illnesses. In 2016 I decided to attend the Health Coach Institute to become a certified health coach, and it is my way of giving back.

What steps have you taken to living your best health? I have eliminated gluten and have added in fun activities as my exercise and social outlet. I have a list of go-to restaurants for social settings because most everybody likes to meet over a meal. I make it a priority to drink purified water and get some sunshine and fresh air when possible. Additionally, I take nutritional supplements when it makes sense.

The one thing that has made the most impact on my heath was to eliminate gluten as a result of doing the elimination diet. Not only did I learn that gluten was an irritant, but also that tomatoes were another major factor that contributed to my painful bladder issues. My interest started with learning what was going on in my body and why, then I addressed my willingness to make some major lifestyle choices to support the needs of my body. I have also made a commitment to stick to my decisions, which is having a positive effect on my health and my life.

My turning point was when I felt like my body hated me. I wasn't able to enjoy life the way I knew I should. Having sinus surgery twice has had a big impact on me, and I had to find a solution so it wouldn't happen again. I had come to the end of the trial prescriptions and the depression they caused. Fortunately, I went to a specialist for the bladder pains who recommended a strict elimination diet. I had no idea at the time what that experiment would unveil for me ... wow!

It's not as hard as it sounds to eat nutritiously, and the payoff may just be that you love your life again. I believe that food is indeed our medicine and that we are as individual as our DNA strands. To assume that we all tolerate all kinds of food just doesn't make any sense. My commitment to better health has changed my life, and living a healthy lifestyle could change yours as well.

> If you can dream it,
> you can achieve it.

Zig Ziglar

Holly Kelsey

Certified Health Coach
www.hollyscoaching.com
holly@hollyscoaching.com

TROPICAL CHEESECAKE

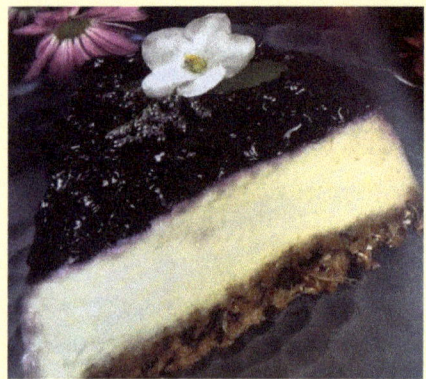

	Per slice
Calories	284
Protein	5g
CHO	59g
Fat	3g
Sugar	36g
Sodium	81mg
Fiber	6g
Chol	0mg

Serves 9

INGREDIENTS

Crust:
- ¾ cup pitted dates chopped
- ¼ cup water
- ¾ cup grape-nuts cereal
- ½ cup quick oats
- 3 tablespoons almonds, finely chopped

Topping:
- 1 ½ cups frozen blueberries or strawberries
- ⅓ cup water
- 2 tablespoons cornstarch

Filling:
- 2 cups tofu, silken, firm (lite)
- 1 tablespoon lemon juice
- 1 tablespoon vanilla
- 1 can pineapple, crushed (do not drain off juice)
- 3 tablespoons cornstarch
- 1 medium banana, peeled and cut into thirds
- ⅓ cup honey

DIRECTIONS

Bring dates and water to boil. Reduce heat to low and simmer, covered, 5 minutes or until soft. Add remaining crust ingredients to date mixture. Mix well. Press mixture into the bottom of a lightly oil-sprayed 9-inch springform pan. Set aside.

Place tofu, lemon juice, vanilla, and half of pineapple into a blender. Blend until very smooth. Pour into a bowl. Place the remaining pineapple, cornstarch, banana, and honey in blender and blend until very smooth. Pour into bowl with other half of mixture. Mix together well. Pour mixture over crust.

Bake at 350°F for approximately 45 minutes, or until edge of cake is browned slightly and center is firm. Cool to room temperature.

In a small pot, mix together frozen berries, water, and cornstarch. Cook over medium heat, stirring constantly, until it has thickened and is clear in color. Spread fruit mixture over the top of the cheesecake. Chill before serving. Slice into 9 pieces.

Chef's Note: Garnish each slice with a fresh mint leaf and berry. For a more tropical taste, substitute frozen mango slices or pineapple pieces in place of the blueberry or strawberry topping.

HUMMUS

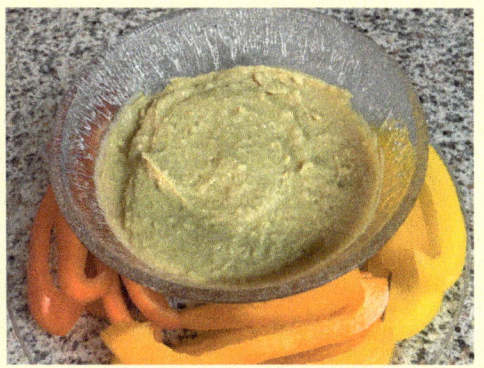

Calories	86
Protein	4g
CHO	13g
Fat	2g
Sugar	1g
Sodium	5mg
Fiber	4g
Chol	0mg

Makes 2 cups

Per ¼ cup serving

INGREDIENTS

- 2 cups garbanzo beans, cooked
- 1 teaspoon tahini (sesame butter)
- 1 teaspoon sesame oil
- 1 ½ tablespoons lemon juice
- ¼ cup parsley, chopped
- ¼ teaspoon garlic powder
- ¼ cup green onions, chopped
- ½ cup green bell peppers, seeded and chopped

DIRECTIONS

Place all ingredients into a blender and blend until smooth. Add additional tahini butter as needed to make a thick spread.

Serve on toast or use as a dip for your favorite raw vegetables.

A NEW LEASE ON LIFE

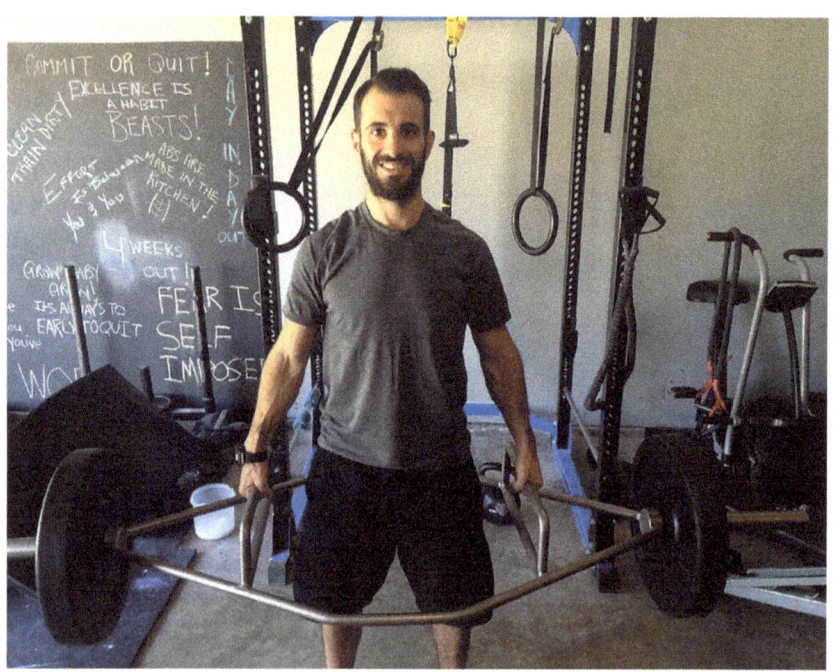

Dan Ferrato

I grew up in Port Coquitlam, British Columbia. Growing up was awesome. I have amazing parents, a very supportive brother, and great friends. My childhood was typical, spending most of my days outside playing with my friends, not having a worry in the world. However, my eating habits weren't the best; in fact, they were very poor. I came from a very Italian household, where any emotion was shown through foods. Whether you were happy, sad, or upset, you ate. Food was always at the forefront. This affected my life in a major way as I was very overweight throughout my entire adolescence, and I grew up as "the fat kid," which still has an effect on me today.

Over the years, I have made some significant changes to those habits. When I was eighteen, my best friend was killed in a motorcycle accident, which led me to choose a career in paramedics. I had to get myself in shape in order to perform the physical assessments required to be a paramedic. At first, I changed everything about my diet and focused on how many calories I was eating and how many calories I was burning. As I learned more about exercise and nutrition, I started filling up those calories with the right types of food, which made all the difference in the world.

My eating habits now play a pivotal role in my life. I have managed to maintain my weight loss of sixty pounds for over twelve years, which has inspired me to become a nutritionist and fitness coach so I can help people slowly change their lives through lifestyle changes. Exercise and nutrition have completely changed my life, and I want to pass this message on to as many people as I can.

I am continuously learning and educating myself in health and fitness. I first became a personal trainer. Next, I became a nutritionist and opened my own fitness business to help inspire others to live a healthy and active life. The loss of my best friend at eighteen was a turning point for another reason, and it led to a major decision I have made that has affected my life in a positive way—being more intentional with whom I surround myself with and whom I choose as my friends.

What is important for me today, and what I value most to pass on to others, is to take life one day at a time and slow down in the process. Don't expect rapid change overnight. Slowly introduce one new habit into your life until it becomes a permanent lifestyle change. Doing this over and over again is the key to long-term success.

> Keep your head in the clouds and feet on the ground.
>
> **Author Unknown**

Dan Ferrato

BCRPA Personal Trainer
FMS Level 1
Precision Nutrition Level 1
www.sweatlab.ca

EGG WHITE FRITTATA

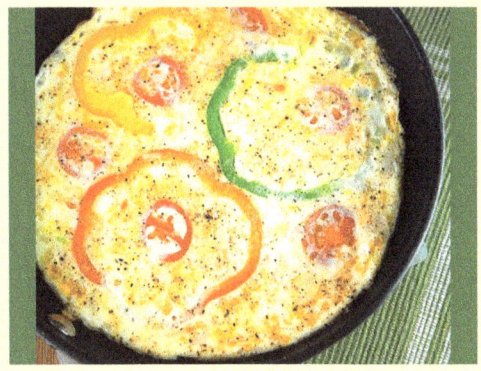

Calories	55
Protein	8g
CHO	5g
Fat	0g
Sugar	2g
Sodium	199mg
Fiber	1g
Chol	0mg

Serves 4

Per serving

INGREDIENTS

- 8 egg whites (1 cup)
- ½ red or green bell pepper, deseeded and sliced
- 3 mushrooms
- ¼ cup purple onion, sliced into slivers
- ½ cup banana peppers, sliced
- 1 clove garlic
- pinch of paprika
- ¼ cup of salsa

DIRECTIONS

Preheat oven to 350°F.

Mix all ingredients and pour into large oiled skillet, then place whole skillet in oven.

Bake at 350°F for 15 minutes.

Chef's note: The egg whites provide a source of protein without adding in additional fats that a whole egg has (although the fats can be good). The vegetables add in additional sources of micronutrients, which will aid in absorption and regular function of the cells inside your body. Along with absorption, the veggies will give you an excellent source of fiber, which will help aid in GI (gastrointestinal) health. GI health is often overlooked when it comes to most people's diets. The addition of salsa and paprika gives the frittata some extra "flare."

POST WORKOUT PROTEIN SHAKE

Makes one shake

INGREDIENTS

- 1 cup filtered water
- 1 scoop of protein powder (any flavor)
- 2 tablespoons ground flaxseed
- ¼–½ cup of steel cut oats
- 1 cup blueberries
- 4–8 ice cubes (depending on how thick you want your shake)

Calories	193
Protein	31g
CHO	15g
Fat	1g
Sugar	8g
Sodium	350mg
Fiber	4g
Chol	0mg

per shake

DIRECTIONS

Place filtered water, protein powder, flax seed, steel cut oats, blueberries, and ice cubes in blender. Blend until shake consistency and place in your favorite work out container.

Chef's note: The protein powder can be whey if you are able to digest it, or a source of hemp protein is excellent as well. After a workout, the body craves fuel (food). In particular, protein and fast-digesting carbohydrates. This shake utilizes liquid protein, which helps the body digest protein at a quicker rate. This will, in turn, help with recovery from an activity. The steel cut oats and blueberries act as a great source of quicker digesting carbohydrates, helping to aid in absorption and help with muscle recovery. Not only that, but the oats and blueberries are another great source of fiber, with the blueberries being high in antioxidants to boot. The flaxseed acts almost as a neutralizer for folks who don't tolerate carbohydrates very well. The flaxseed can help slow the rate of digestion of the carbs without limiting the amount of carbohydrates needed. Flaxseed is also an amazing source of omega-3s, which help with joint recovery and everything else in your body.

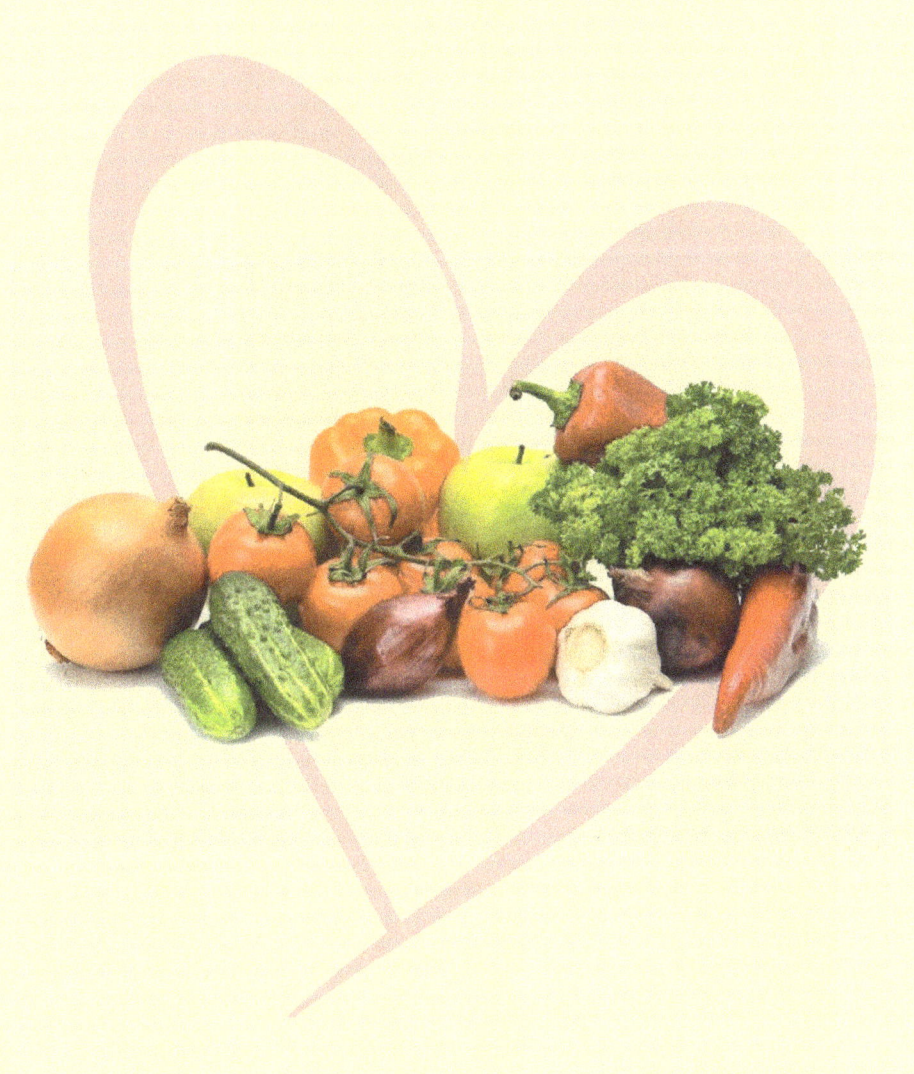

THE POWER OF FOOD

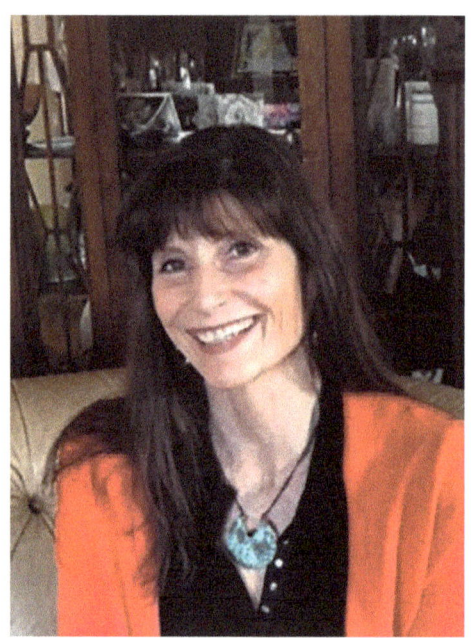

Dana Camera

I grew up in Long Beach, New York, which was a great place to grow up—especially in the summer! I was the change-of-life baby for my family, special from the start. I was born on my mother's forty-fifth birthday, my dad had just turned forty-nine, and my three sisters were age eighteen, sixteen, and thirteen. Surprise was an understatement!

Due to the fact that my sisters were much older, I grew up like an only child. I'm fiercely independent, and alone time is a necessity in my life.

I am also Italian American, and this is a prerequisite for loving food! My mom was an excellent and healthy cook, and she prepared our meals daily for us. Going out to eat at a restaurant was a rare treat.

My journey with food started at a young age. When I was ten years old, I walked into my pediatrician's office, and he told me that I was fat. This one statement caused food obsession, low self-esteem, poor body image and a dysfunctional relationship to food. This led to thirty-five years of yo-yo dieting. Point being, if there was a diet out there, I've tried it, thinking that this was the answer to inner peace. The good news is that I've figured out the mystery of sustainable weight loss.

I started working part-time in a pizzeria while going to community college full-time. I was eating pizza, pasta, fried foods, and drinking soda. This one job in my life led to severe weight gain and fed the yo-yo dieting syndrome even further. In 1996, I was diagnosed with Crohn's disease, which led to surgery within three months after diagnosis, another three years later, and nine years after that. After using conventional medicine, I was on countless medications for years. I realized that I was just existing and not thriving.

My turning point came in 2004, when I finally learned the power of food. I had changed my diet drastically overnight with the help of two women who were chemical molecular biologists, referred to me by my sister. I learned how to cook and eat new foods. This was not an easy time for me; however, I stuck to it. The payoff? My blood work was normal within nine weeks of changing my diet, and my blood work hadn't been normal in eight years after my diagnosis. I was truly amazed! Due to a holistic approach to food and lifestyle, I haven't dealt with symptoms of Crohn's disease for over a decade.

In 2012, I was diagnosed with Acute Myeloid Leukemia (AML)—a shocker! I was confused, scared, and a little angry, because I thought I was doing everything right. I was in the hospital for five months with two short breaks. I had five rounds of chemotherapy (which almost damaged my body beyond repair) and a stem cell transplant (which saved my life; my sister was a 100 percent match). My diet had slipped off the straight and narrow after that. Then, three months after getting out of the hospital, super storm Sandy hit us. The stress that followed was extreme, and we lost our home. My immune system took a huge hit. The first two years after my transplant, I was getting weird infections every few months. It seemed never-ending. The reason why I'm still here to talk about it is because my nutritionist said, "Dana, you know what to do to heal yourself." I then implemented the tools I had been taught, one day at a time, until I got my life back! I cannot say enough about the power of food and lifestyle management.

I've chosen to be a health coach because my passion is to help others take control of their lives. Let's be honest: I've been through the ringer when it comes to my health. Many times, I was at a dead end and I didn't know how to approach sustainable healing. I now choose to live well. Every time I eat something, I say to myself, "Does this serve me?" This is a powerful statement, and makes me think before I put just anything into my mouth. I do have my days when I'm running on empty and my choices feed my brain, but not my body! Those days occur less frequently as I'm learning and evolving.

Over the last twenty-one years, I have learned that food is medicine. I maintain a lifestyle of eating well 80–90 percent of the time and having small indulgences 10–20 percent of the time. Through trial and error, I've learned what types of food gives me energy, helps stabilize my mood, and agrees with my system. I've become more mindful of what I'm putting into my body. I focus on what I *can* eat, instead of what I choose not to eat. I now think of my body as a luxury car. The car runs on a certain fuel, and if the fuel is not right for the engine, the car will run poorly—or not at all.

In conclusion, I know my story is extraordinary. The statement, "You are what you eat," is truth. The food that is promoted in grocery stores, commercials, and billboards will slowly kill you. The keys to a healthy life are water, whole foods, stress management, movement, connecting to others, sleep, self-love, and respect. My goal is to let the people that cross my path know about the power of food. You didn't gain weight overnight, nor did you get sick overnight; there is no quick fix. Small, steady changes last a lifetime and lead to undeniable health!

> **Small, steady changes last a lifetime.**

Dana Camera

Certified Holistic Health Coach
Long Beach, NY
danajcamera@gmail.com
www.danacamera.com

CHIA PORRIDGE

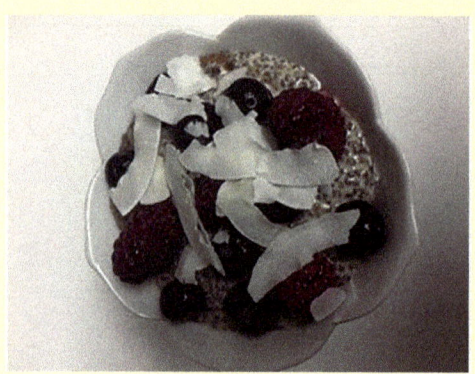

Serves 4

Calories	230
Protein	7g
CHO	35g
Fat	8g
Sugar	8g
Sodium	81mg
Fiber	21g
Chol	0mg

Per serving *Nutritional information does not include garnish

INGREDIENTS

- ½ cup chia seeds
- 1 teaspoon vanilla
- 1 tablespoon cinnamon
- 4 dates, pitted and chopped
- 16 ounces nut milk
- berries, cacao nibs, or nuts for garnish*

DIRECTIONS

Combine chia seeds, vanilla, and cinnamon. Then, chop the dates and add to the bowl. Add nut milk. Cover bowl, and let it sit overnight in the refrigerator. Garnish with fresh berries, cacao nibs, or nuts. Enjoy!

BEAN BURGERS

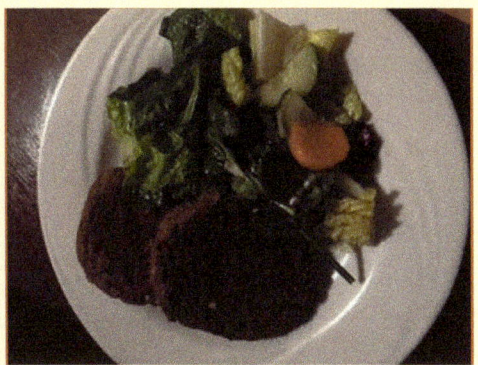

Calories	470
Protein	19g
CHO	67g
Fat	17g
Sugar	3g
Sodium	346mg
Fiber	15g
Chol	0mg

Serves 4

Per serving

INGREDIENTS

- 1 can organic beans (your choice), rinsed and drained
- ¼ cup walnuts
- ¼ medium yellow onion, diced
- ½ large zucchini, diced
- ¼ cup gluten-free bread crumbs
- ¼ cup ground flax seed
- 2 tablespoons avocado oil
- 1 tablespoon grated pecorino Romano cheese (optional)
- 1 tablespoon parsley
- ½ teaspoon garlic powder
- ½ teaspoon paprika
- ½ teaspoon Himalayan sea salt
- ½ teaspoon black pepper

DIRECTIONS

Preheat oven to 400°F. Put all ingredients in the food processor. Form into patties. Bake in the oven on parchment paper at 400°F, for 6–7 minutes on each side or until golden brown. Alternatively, you can cook these in a skillet over medium heat, sprayed with cooking spray, 6–7 minutes on each side or until golden brown. Again, this is a versatile recipe, so add what you like and keep the measurements the same.

FOR THE LOVE OF FOOD

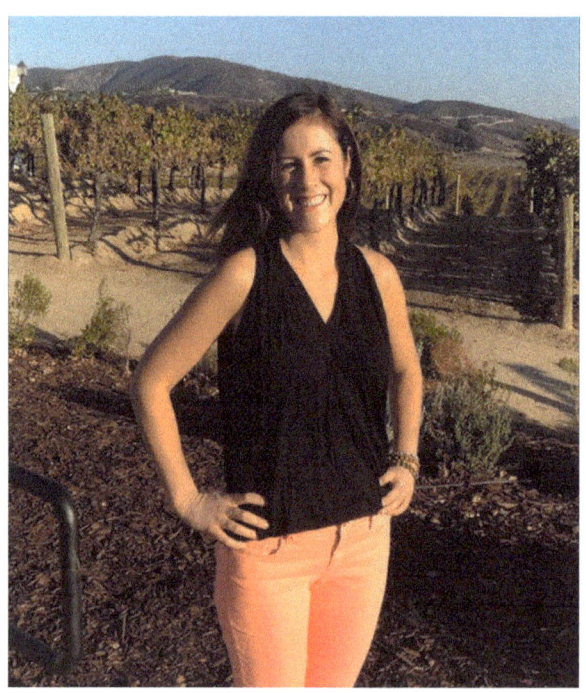

Jessica Geist

As a dietitian, I find myself straying from the word "diet" quite frequently. I believe many dietitians can agree that diets don't work and that finding happiness with one's self comes from balance. That is what I have been trying to communicate over the various paths my career has taken thus far in the dietetics field. I am a lover of food. A meal is so much more than a means of nourishment. It is a feeling of comfort and love. A specific taste can bring us back to a memory and fill us with joy.

In an interview, I was once asked such a wonderful question that it has continued to remain with me. I was asked to name a dish that brings about a favorite memory. My answer was homemade raviolis. Although not the healthiest, these are made from scratch using real, whole ingredients. The process happens once a year prior to Christmas dinner where they are frozen and saved for the big day. Over the years, my Nana has passed her specific ravioli making process down through the generations. The day is long, and it can be gruelling to prepare enough for a large crowd. There are usually frustrations, and my Nana is never quite content with our work as she oversees the preparation. The day, however, always ends in laughs and great memories for us and other family members who stop in to assist. Sharing them on Christmas Day with all of the people who mean the most to me inspires an overwhelming feeling of joy that I look forward to year after year.

My hope as a dietitian is to help others truly enjoy food. Food should not be a source of fear. We should embrace real ingredients and take the time to prepare meals from scratch. Although cooking can seem daunting in today's hectic environment, recipes can be simple and healthy. Taking time to cook together can bring families closer together and help to slow down the daily rush.

My passion for helping others embrace the power of food has led me to a career in dietetics. Volunteer work helping food bank recipients learn how to make healthy, simple, low-cost meals with their families was a rewarding and eye-opening experience. It amazed me to see what people can do with food once you give them the tools to recreate healthy meals at home. This inspired me to pursue a major in nutrition and management at the University of Massachusetts Amherst and further my dietetics career through an internship with the University of New Hampshire.

My first position as an R.D.N. was with a small hospital as a temporary dietitian in Nome, Alaska, where I worked with a native population. I gained experience as both an inpatient and outpatient dietitian. I provided community outreach through health fairs throughout neighboring villages and taking part as an educator in the Diabetes Prevention Program.

After returning to Massachusetts, I decided I wanted to let my career lead me on yet another adventure. I landed a job in Hemet, California, as a clinical dietitian. I quickly worked my way to lead dietitian in the ICU department, helping to nourish critically ill patients with various disease states. Although this was a rewarding career, I wanted to work closer with food. An opportunity opened for a general manager position in our sister hospital where I am currently training as an interim general manager to gain the experience necessary to fill this role.

I hope to further my career by helping others find a healthy relationship with food. Creating healthy, balanced meals at home with whole ingredients can do so much more than help nourish our bodies to help protect against chronic disease. Cooking at home can help spark creativity when playing with different ingredients and new flavors. It can bring us closer to family by getting them involved in meal preparation and sit-down dinners. It can also be a source of relaxation, knowing we are preparing quality meals to serve to the ones we love. I hope my involvement in this cookbook helps guide others to embrace food, rather than be afraid of it, since food will always be my first love.

> The purpose of life is to live it,
> to taste experience to the utmost,
> to reach out eagerly and without fear
> for newer and richer experience.
>
> **Eleanor Roosevelt**

Jessica Geist, RDN

Wareham, Massachusetts
jmgeist71@gmail.com

ITALIAN BAKED HADDOCK

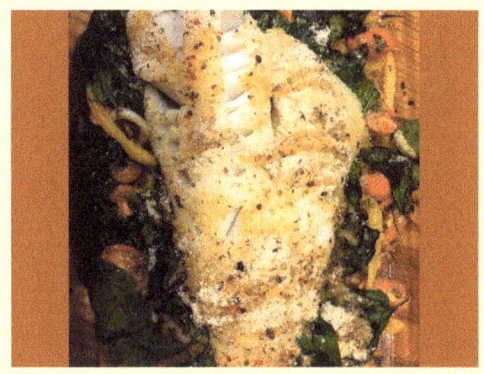

Calories	219
Protein	23g
CHO	14g
Fat	8g
Sugar	3g
Sodium	125mg
Fiber	2g
Chol	49mg

Serves 4   Per serving

INGREDIENTS

- 1 pound Atlantic caught cod or halibut
- 2 tablespoons olive oil + extra for drizzling
- 1 cup grape tomatoes, halved
- 2 cloves garlic, finely chopped
- 2 teaspoons fresh parsley
- 4 tablespoons plain breadcrumbs or gluten-free bread crumbs
- 1 teaspoon oregano
- ¼ teaspoon crushed red pepper flakes
- ½ cup orange bell pepper, thinly sliced
- ½ cup yellow bell pepper, thinly sliced
- ½ cup shallots, thinly sliced
- 2 cups baby spinach
- salt and pepper to taste

DIRECTIONS

Preheat oven to 375°F.

In a medium-sized bowl, combine 2 tablespoons olive oil, tomatoes, garlic, parsley, peppers, shallots, salt and pepper to taste. Toss well.

In a small bowl, combine bread crumbs, oregano, red pepper flakes.

Spray 9 x13 inch baking dish with cooking spray or coat with olive oil. Sprinkle 2 tablespoons bread crumb mixture over pan. Cover with vegetable mixture. Bake for 15 minutes.

Cover vegetable mixture with 2 cups baby spinach. Rinse fish and pat dry with a paper towel. Place fish on top of vegetables. Sprinkle fish with salt and pepper to taste. Drizzle good amount of olive oil over fish and vegetables. Bake for 25 minutes until fish is opaque and flaky.

RUSTIC MUSHROOM POLENTA

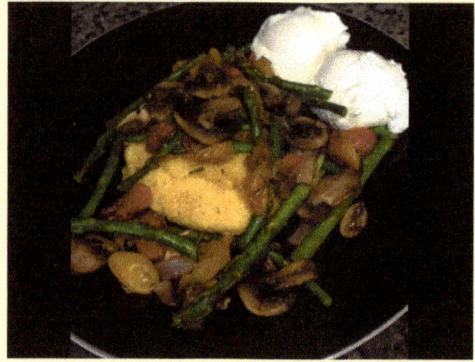

Calories	221
Protein	6g
CHO	32g
Fat	18g
Sugar	4g
Sodium	167mg
Fiber	4g
Chol	4mg

Serves 4   Per serving

INGREDIENTS

- 1 ½ cups low sodium vegetable stock
- 1 ½ cups water
- olive oil to coat pan
- 2 cloves of garlic, finely chopped
- 1 large shallot, sliced
- 3 cups assorted Baby Bella, cremini, or white mushrooms, sliced
- 1 cup grape tomatoes, halved
- ½ of one bunch thin asparagus
- ¾ teaspoon fresh rosemary, chopped
- ¼ teaspoon fresh thyme
- 1 tablespoon balsamic vinegar
- salt and pepper to taste
- 1 cup dry polenta (corn grits)
- 3 tablespoons pecorino Romano cheese, shaved or grated
- 1 tablespoon white vinegar, optional

DIRECTIONS

Bring water and vegetable stock to a boil.

In the meantime, heat olive oil over medium heat. Add shallots and garlic, stirring frequently until fragrant. Add tomatoes, mushrooms, and asparagus. Cook for about 10 minutes until soft. Add rosemary and thyme and heat for another two minutes. Drizzle with balsamic vinegar. Season with salt and pepper to taste. Remove from heat.

Stir polenta slowly into boiling water and reduce heat to low. Add cheese if using and stir until melted through. Cook through for 5 minutes. Cover and remove from heat to let thicken for another 2 minutes.

To plate, place ¼ prepared polenta on plate. Top with heaping cup of sautéed vegetables.

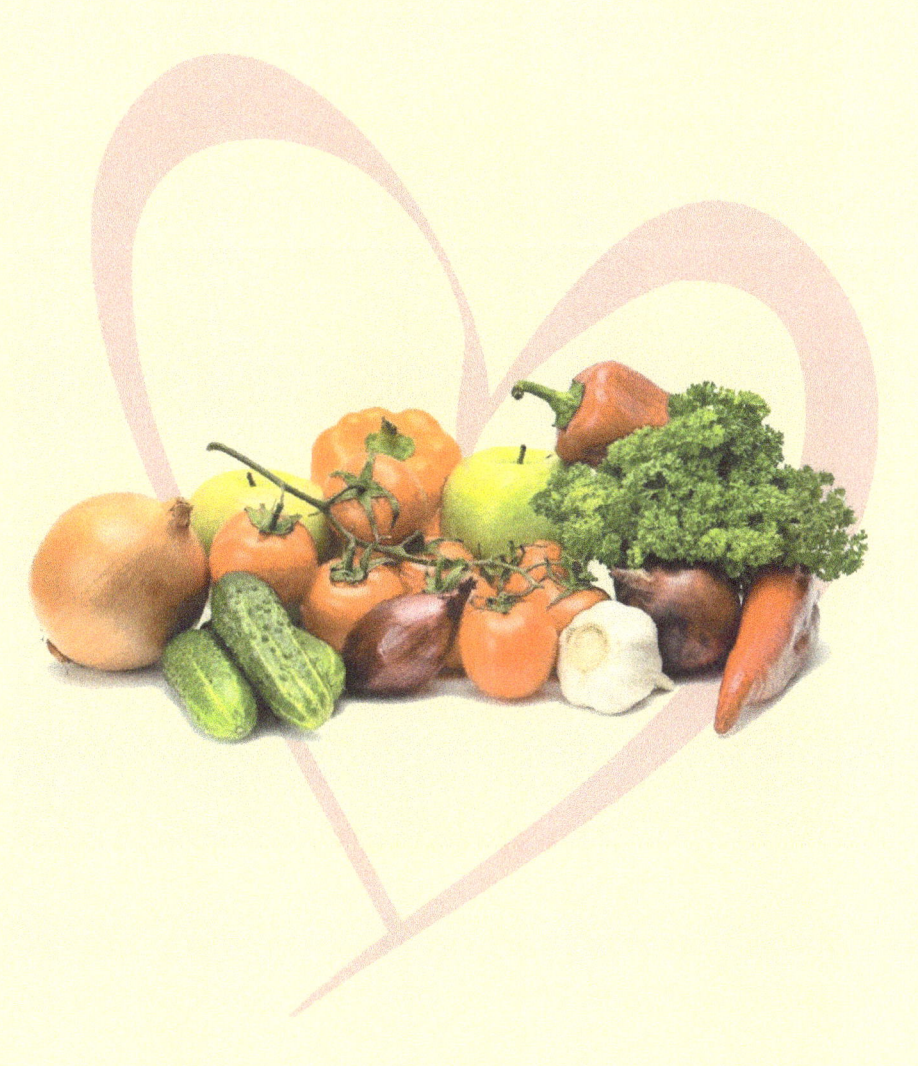

HEALTH IS OUR MOST IMPORTANT ASSET

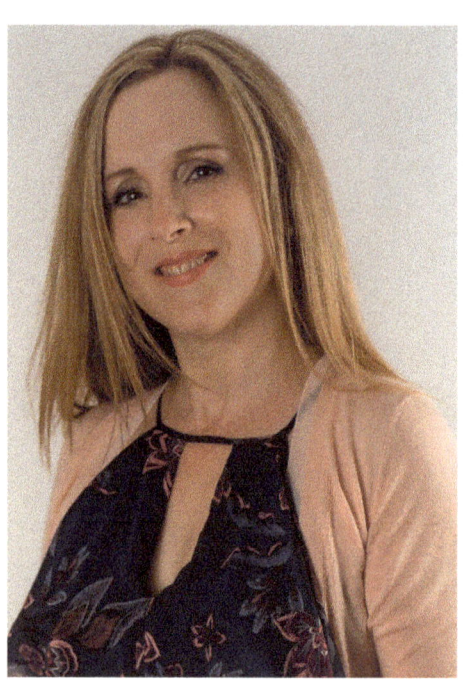

Lucie Woods

I am grateful for the work that Linda and Joyce are doing, as it is time to share and educate the world on what matters most in our life: our health. Health is our most important asset, and we have the power to make choices around our health so that we live a healthy, vibrant life.

I grew up in a small town called Sherbrook in the province of Quebec. Like most children, my life was to play, eat, and go to school. I remember going out daily with my youngest sister to visit my three elder neighbors to find out what they had in their backyard. To our excitement and surprise, we discovered that they had a tremendous vegetable garden with fresh tomatoes, cucumbers, lettuce, and much more. My sister and I got into the habit of visiting and asking for cucumbers, as they tasted so fresh, crunchy, and delicious. Those days spending time with these elder ladies, talking for hours and learning from their wisdom, were a great treat for us.

Some forty years ago, I recall eating anything that was available without any concern for nutritional value: white bread, cakes, cookies, some fruits, raw vegetables, cheese, meat, potatoes, etc. That is how I was raised. I did not question what I ate. I felt I was safe, healthy, and I did not have the thought process that I have today. Now that I am responsible for my children and their health and what they should or should not eat, when I go to the grocery store, I pay attention to the ingredients by reading labels to make sure I feed myself and my family with the best ingredients possible.

My interest toward food today is the reality that the nutritional value is not what it was forty to sixty years ago. I realized this when I was diagnosed with a low thyroid issue. My doctor said that I had to take medication for my thyroid. I asked if I would have to take this for the rest of my life, and his response was yes. Then my arms dropped, and I said to him that would never happen. I knew then that I would have to figure this out by myself.

I thought there was something to contribute to this condition, so I decided to find out what that might be. I also decided that it was time to make some lifestyle changes that might help. I began to research what causes low thyroid issue, and adrenal fatigue as it relates to a thyroid problem. My symptoms were fatigue, mood swings, and low energy, to mention a few.

When you are ready to make changes, life brings what you need, and

I was referred to a naturopath who completed blood tests so we could get to the bottom of the problem. I also started to add supplements to my diet hoping they would help. I changed my diet to give my body the nutrients that it needed to get back to a place of feeling healthy and remaining healthy.

By changing my diet, taking the right supplements, exercising, and being more conscious of breathing, plus natural medication, I was able to get the hypothyroid issue back to normal functioning within twelve months. This was a different scenario than what my physician proposed at first with lifetime medication.

But that was not the turning point for me. A few years prior to this event, I discovered that my first child was hyperactive, had uncontrollable temper tantrums, signs of ADHD, and more. I knew that something was going on with my health, but first I had to figure out what was going on with my daughter. She was one of those kids with sensory processing disorders, which include all the above signs. That was the big wakeup call of my life to learn how to support her and find out what was going on with me. After a few years, she was diagnosed with candida, which is a yeast imbalance in the intestinal flora that can be caused by antibiotics and diet. In fact, high sugar in diet can weaken the immune system, resulting in candida infection. I read that candida is often found in children with autism. We are now on a sugar-free diet, no gluten, no dairy. She takes minerals and supplements that were missing in her body and eating a more balance nutritious diet. We have observed dramatic changes in her mood levels, fewer temper tantrums, and she is more joyful and sociable.

I cannot explain in just a few words how important nutrition is, how it affects us, or the numerous benefits our body will receive. Hopefully my short story will explain how the simple changes we made to a healthier lifestyle have transformed our health and life forever. By adding light physical exercise, breathing techniques, and vitamin and mineral supplements, we have helped to reduce stress levels, mood swings, improve metabolisms, bowel movements, and much more. Nutrition, in my opinion, is the number one key to rejuvenate and nourish our bodies.

While on this journey, I thought I was not alone with these types of conditions. However, after reading the statistics about how sick people are today with heart diseases, adrenal fatigues, thyroid problems, autism, dementia, cancer, and more, I decided to bring my contribution to this world by becoming a certified health coach. I can now help and educate people and families just like mine about health and nutrition, so they can live a long, healthy, and happy life. Let's be the change!

> Believe you can and you are halfway there.
>
> **President Roosevelt**

Lucie Woods, Conscious Healthy Lives

Certified Health Coach
Coquitlam, British Columbia
www.conscioushealthylives.com
info@conscioushealthylives.com

TUNA & AVOCADO SALAD

Serves 2

INGREDIENTS

- 1 (12 ounce) can low sodium albacore tuna in water
- 1 full avocado (medium size), cut in pieces
- 1 small pack of cherry tomatoes, sliced

FRESH HOMADE DRESSING

- 1 tablespoon fresh squeezed lemon
- fresh basil and/or oregano to taste

DIRECTIONS

Combine all ingredients together and mix with the salad dressing. Delicious as a meal, as a snack, and as a sandwich with gluten-free bread.

Calories	322
Protein	47g
CHO	5g
Fat	13g
Sugar	2g
Sodium	120mg
Fiber	6g
Chol	67mg

Per serving

CHICKEN & APPLE SANDWICH

Makes 2 servings

INGREDIENTS

- 1 cup of cooked organic free-range chicken breast, cubed
- ¼ cup celery, diced
- ¼ cup apple (your choice), diced
- 1 tablespoon avocado oil mayonnaise (non-GMO, soy free)
- pinch of Himalayan salt

DIRECTIONS

Prepare chicken ahead of time and place in refrigerator until ready to use. Toss everything together lightly, until combined. Add the mix to gluten-free quinoa bread or use to top a green salad.

Calories	154
Protein	22g
CHO	4g
Fat	5g
Sugar	4g
Sodium	188mg
Fiber	0g
Chol	65mg

Per serving (does not include bread)

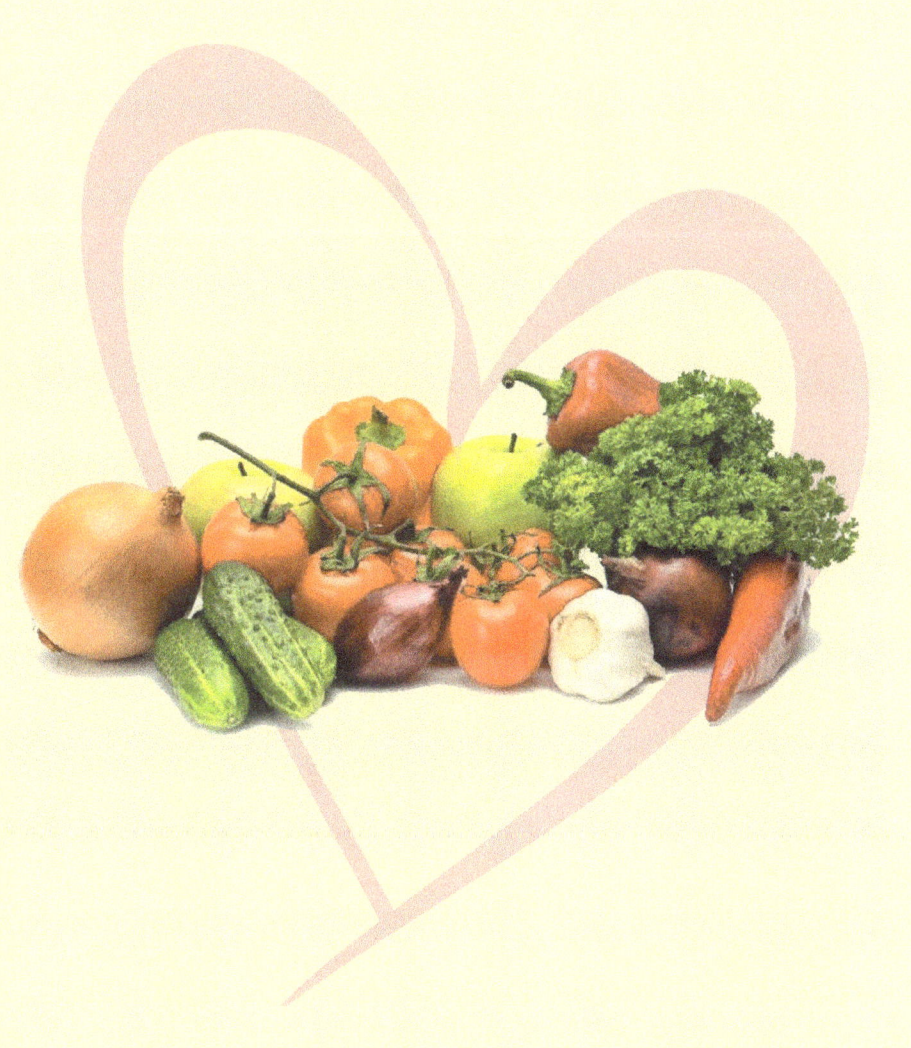

FOOD IS FOOD

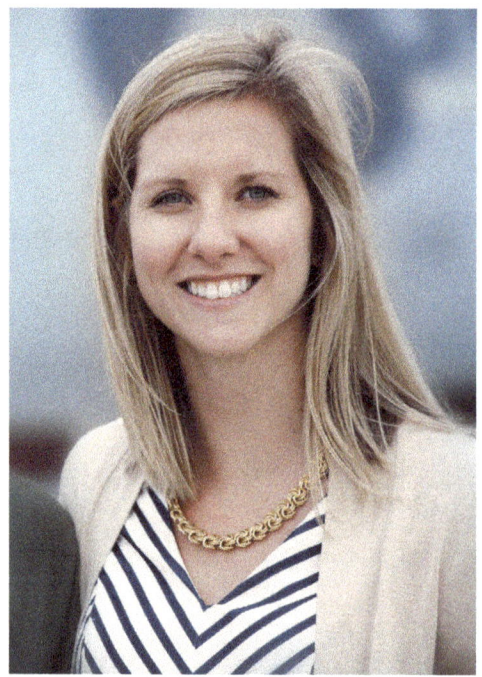

Laura Stempky

I was born in the small town of Cheboygan, Michigan, and grew up in the suburbs of Cincinnati, Ohio. I spent my early years of life with what I would call now a normal, healthy relationship with food: eating what I wanted, when I wanted, without feeling guilty. I grew up in a food-loving family. While that meant I ate plenty of processed and fast food, my family also had a huge vegetable garden that I spent many summer days perusing. Looking back at that time, it was the perfect balance:

plenty of fresh fruits and vegetables with an indulgent treat every now and then. I listened to my body and gave it the fuel it needed.

However, for reasons unbeknownst to me, but likely influenced by the society at large, I started restricting my diet and exercising obsessively in my early teenage years. I only ate reduced fat or sugar-free foods. I felt guilty every time I ate a cookie. I cried if I missed an exercise session. I tracked my weight every day. This lasted two years, which included doctor appointments for missed menstruation, heated and defensive conversations with friends and family, an overall poor self-image, and even poorer self-confidence.

One day I finally had enough. I was sick of that restricted and regimented lifestyle that permeated the rest of my life. I clearly recall my life-changing decision. I was eating a handful of Teddy Grahams and remember thinking, *I can eat these and feel guilty because they have sugar in them, or I can eat these because they taste good and they are what my body wants right now*. I decided on the latter. I was able to snap out of that life relatively quickly, for which I am grateful. That is not to say it was easy or that I do not struggle with feelings of guilt today. It is still a journey, but every day is a little bit easier.

When it was time to go to college and earn a degree, I consistently thought back to my restrictive years and how far I had come. I was cooking often and wanted to learn more about food. I became fascinated with the science behind nutrition and how to cook foods that properly nourish the body.

Fueled with knowledge gained from education, plus my personal experiences with food, I worked as a dietitian in a hospital and in nursing homes. I love the hospital setting because food is such an integral part of healing and prevention of disease. I may only have seen a patient one time before they headed home, or to another facility. However, if I was able to impart one tidbit of knowledge regarding nutrition, I felt like I made a difference.

After three years—and much thought and deliberation—I decided to return to school to become a registered nurse. I realized I wanted to advance my knowledge of the body, how it works, and further ways to prevent disease. I recently received my RN degree, and I am excited to be able to spend more time with patients to continue to spread my passion of nutrition.

My lifestyle and eating habits have come a long way from my youth. While inspired by different stages of my life, my relationship with food is the best it has been. My current motto: Food is food. It is meant to nourish our bodies and give them the fuel they need to live a happy, active life. "Bad" foods do not exist; "good" foods do not exist. There are some foods that better nourish the body, but there are other foods that better nourish the soul. The conscious decision to think this way has made the most positive impact on my health and life overall.

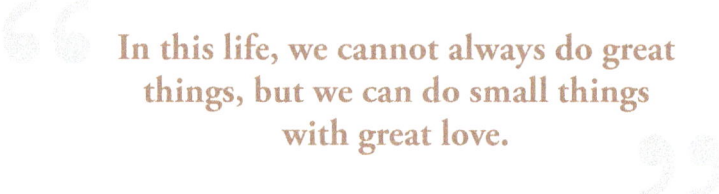

In this life, we cannot always do great things, but we can do small things with great love.

Mother Teresa

Laura Stempky, BSN, RDN

West Chester, Ohio
lkstempky@gmail.com

STUFFED SWEET POTATOES

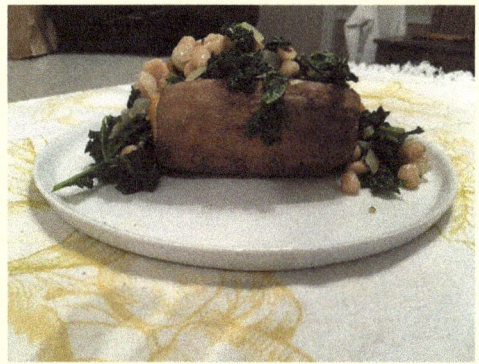

Calories	344
Protein	11g
CHO	59g
Fat	7g
Sugar	13g
Sodium	171mg
Fiber	13g
Chol	0mg

Serves 4

Per serving

INGREDIENTS

- 4 whole sweet potatoes, cleaned
- 2 tablespoons olive oil
- 1 shallot, diced (I often use one small onion.)
- 2 garlic cloves, minced
- 1 (4-inch) sprig fresh rosemary
- ¼ teaspoon red pepper flakes (add more or less depending on spiciness desired)
- 1 ½ cups (or one 15 ounce can) cooked and drained white beans (cannellini)
- 6 cups kale, trimmed and sliced into ribbons
- juice of ¼ lemon
- salt and freshly ground black pepper

DIRECTIONS

Preheat oven to 400°F.

Clean the sweet potatoes and prick them in a few places with a fork. Wrap in foil and bake until soft, 45 minutes to 1 hour.

With 20 minutes before the sweet potatoes are done, begin cooking the beans and kale.

Heat the olive oil over medium low heat in a wide, deep skillet with a cover. Add the shallots (or onions) and cook until softened, about 5 minutes. Add the garlic, rosemary and red pepper flakes. Cook, stirring constantly until fragrant, about 1 minute. Add the beans and cook for 5 minutes, stirring occasionally. Add the kale to the pan, cover, and cook until kale is soft, about 5 minutes. Remove rosemary sprig and stir in lemon juice. Season with salt and pepper as desired.

When sweet potatoes are soft, allow to cool slightly. Slice each potato in half. Spoon beans and kale into the center.

CREAMED PEAR TOPPING

Makes 4 cups

INGREDIENTS

- ⅓ cup raw cashews
- 1 teaspoon vanilla extract
- 3½ cups (28 ounces) canned pears, unsweetened

DIRECTIONS

Drain juices from canned pears and reserve.

Place all ingredients into a blender, omitting the reserved juice.

Blend until very smooth. Slowly pour juice reserved from pears into a blender as needed until the desired consistency.

Variation: Substitute canned peaches or frozen thawed strawberries for canned pears.

Calories	55
Protein	1g
CHO	8g
Fat	2g
Sugar	5g
Sodium	3mg
Fiber	1g
Chol	0mg

per ¼ cup serving

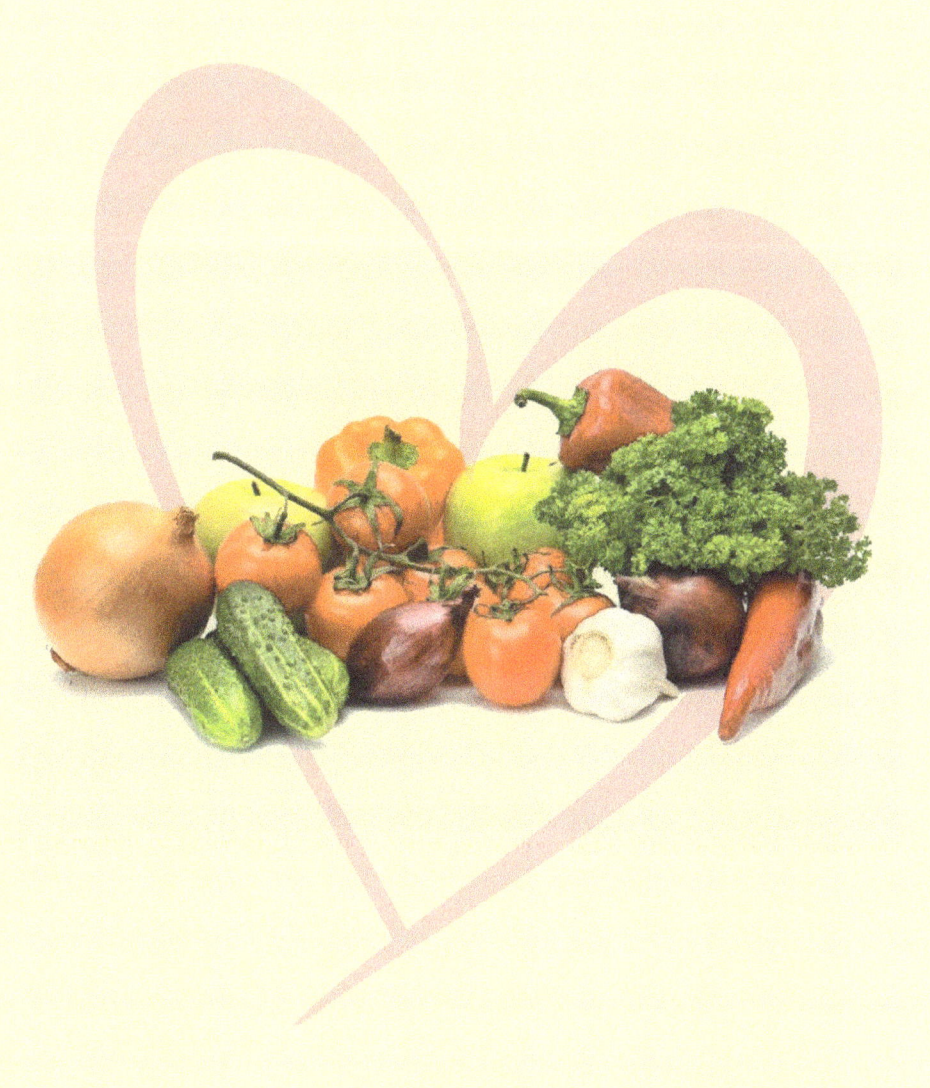

DETERMINED TO BE HEALTHY & FIT

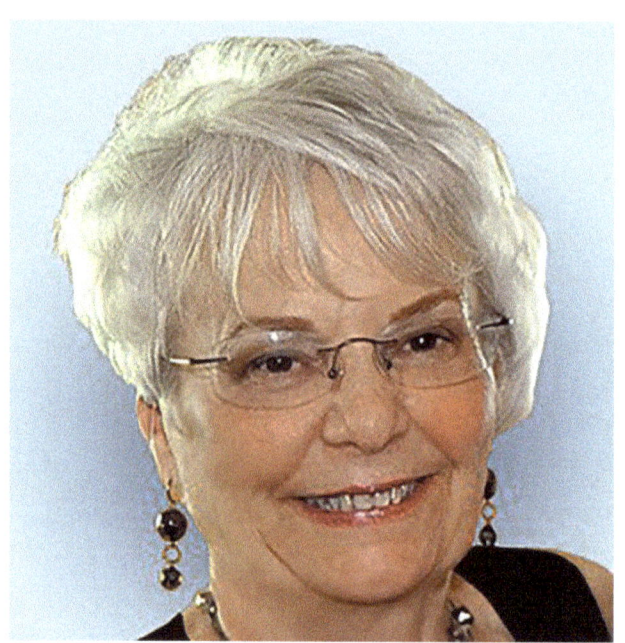

Donna Willon

I grew up in Vancouver, British Columbia—yes, a true Vancouverite. Although I did leave for several years, I decided to make Vancouver my permanent home. As a family, we lived in a basement suite in the house where my grandma and grandpa also lived upstairs.

My grandparents owned a bakery, and my mom worked there. That's how the bread and sweets came into my life. My stepfather was from

England, and that's where the roast beef yorkshire puddings and roasted potatoes smeared with gravy came from. We really thought we were eating well, and of course the aroma when you walked into the house was irresistible. I can still smell that apple pie.

I can now admit that I was a bit of a brat when I was growing up; things bothered me, and I would definitely react to them. However, I never would have put it down to the food we were eating, nor would I contribute food to the lack of energy or enthusiasm I had towards playing many sports. However, now it makes sense; as delicious as the food was, I can now see how it affected me.

In my adult years, I had breast cancer and type 2 diabetes. I was also diagnosed with sleep apnea. That was the last straw; I was not going to wear one of those masks to bed. I questioned what would it take to help me resolve these conditions, and the answer was simple: I needed to lose some weight. Once I did, my diabetes disappeared. As for the cancer, I managed to overcome it gracefully, but it really made me aware that something needed to change. I've lost many of my family to cancer. I am grateful that I am a survivor! I put these health issues down to "stress and the lack of good nutrition," the real, whole-food type.

I tried many diet programs over the years, and every time I lost weight; however, the weight seemed to come back so I would try again. It was a rollercoaster ride during those years and, although I finally found a way to stabilize my weight, I still wasn't feeling the energy and enthusiasm that I wanted. In addition, I started having aches and pains, something I have low tolerance or patience for. I thought to myself, *When is enough? I'm sure I am eating well, so what's wrong?*

That's when I saw several practitioners to get rid of the aches and pains. One practitioner said that my major problem was in my digestive system. I questioned how that could be. I was eating well, or so I thought. My weight was fairly okay, so how could I have a digestive problem? The practitioner told me that I wasn't eating the best foods for my body—real foods. At home, I looked at what I was eating and realized that obviously I didn't know how to choose a good nutritional plan for myself, or my body type, and definitely needed some help.

That's when I decided it was time to hire a health coach to help me design a nutritional plan that would work for me. Working with Linda McLeod, Certified Health & Lifestyle Coach, has been the best decision I have made in years. I'm the type of person that if something is going wrong with me, then tell me how to fix it and I'll do it. Linda has been the support I needed.

I'm now in my seventies. I have two sons, four grandchildren, and a nephew who lost his mom (my sister) to cancer. My mom, dad, step dad, uncle, and grandparents are all gone. I'm now the matriarch of the family, and I want to be an example, not only for myself but also to my family and others as well. My desire is to live as pain free as possible, and to be as healthy as I can so I can have the energy to enjoy my life with friends and family. I'm not giving into disease and aches and pains!

I recently took a step toward improving my life by taking a two-week whole body reset cleanse. I did exactly what I was supposed to, and it made such a positive impact on my health that I have continued on with the food plan. I am slowing introducing some foods that I love, but no sweets or gluten—it has been awesome. My energy is better than it has ever been! My blood pressure is low, my diabetes count is lower than it has ever been, and I sleep solidly … better than a baby.

My life has been transformed. I have cleaned out my cupboards of canned goods, wheat, packages of sauces, gravies, plus all dairies from my fridge. Now I drink decaffeinated teas and my nutritional base is real, whole foods. I have no cravings for foods that I used to eat or drink, and I feel better than ever before. It can be easy if you are really committed to your health. You can make it fun, enjoyable, and turn your health and life into what you want it to be.

So ask yourself, how long and how many years does it take to find out who you are and what is really important to you? Have you ever wondered why you are irritable, cranky, out of sorts, or not feeling as well and energetic as you would like to? Are you concerned about why you are so tired and have a lack of energy? You are the CEO of your health. You are in charge! Don't wait for your crisis. Make a decision to live your abundant life NOW. This is my decision, as it is really important to me and my future health.

> Life isn't about finding yourself.
> Life is about creating yourself.

George Bernard Shaw

Donna Willon

CEO Focused Networking
Coquitlam, BC
www.focusednetworking.com

HALIBUT SKEWERS WITH LIME

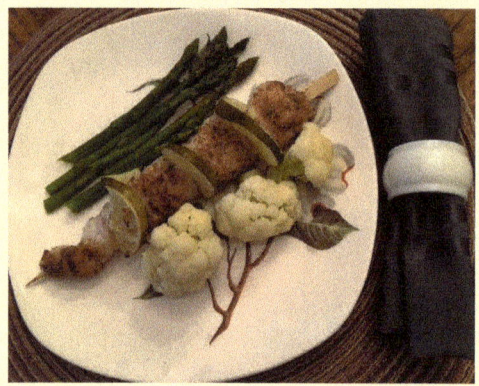

Calories	269
Protein	28g
CHO	6g
Fat	16g
Sugar	1g
Sodium	171mg
Fiber	2g
Chol	65mg

Serves 4

Per serving

INGREDIENTS

- ¾ teaspoon ground cumin
- ¾ teaspoon smoked paprika
- 1 tablespoon chopped fresh oregano
- ¼ teaspoon crushed red pepper flakes
- 3 limes, divided
- 1 ½ pounds boneless, skinless wild-caught Atlantic halibut, cut into 1-inch pieces
- 2 tablespoons olive oil + additional for brushing on grill
- salt to taste

DIRECTIONS

Heat a grill to medium heat.

Combine spices together in a small bowl.

Slice 2 limes very thinly into rounds.

Skewer halibut and lime slices on double-pronged or 2 parallel skewers, beginning and ending with the halibut. Brush halibut with olive oil and sprinkle both sides with reserved spice mixture.

Brush grill with olive oil and grill skewers 2 ½ to 4 minutes on each side, depending on thickness, until fish flakes easily with a fork. Cut remaining lime into 6 wedges and serve with skewers.

Chef's Note: You can also thread cherry tomatoes or super thin ribbons of zucchini with the fish and lime. You can make the spice mixture weeks in advance and keep in a glass jar at room temperature. If you are using the lime slices, don't make the fish skewers more than an hour in advance otherwise the lime will "cook" the fish.

SMOKED SALMON AVOCADO BREAKFAST WITH SIDE DISH YOGURT AND FRUIT

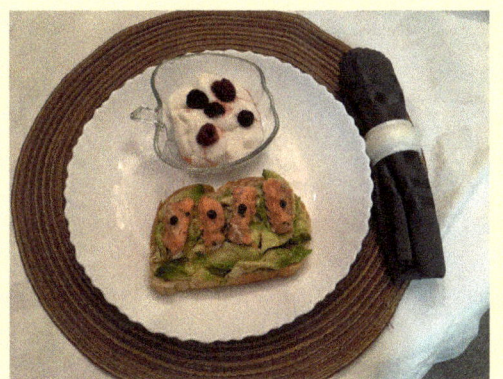

Calories	450
Protein	39g
CHO	54g
Fat	10g
Sugar	28g
Sodium	333mg
Fiber	7g
Chol	23mg

Serves 1

Per serving

INGREDIENTS

Avocado Toast

- 1 slice gluten-free potato bread, toasted
- ¼ cup avocado, mashed
- 2 ounces low-sodium smoked salmon
- ½ teaspoon capers, rinsed, for garnish

Berry Yogurt

- 1 cup nonfat Greek yogurt or soy yogurt of choice
- coconut extract
- ¼ cup fresh coconut, shredded
- ½ cup fresh blueberries

DIRECTIONS

Spread mashed avocado on toasted gluten-free potato bread. Place the smoked salmon over the avocado, then top with capers for garnish.

For the side dish, place yogurt in a small bowl, then sweeten with coconut extract or fresh coconut. Top with blueberries.

CONSTANT PAIN TO GREAT HEALTH

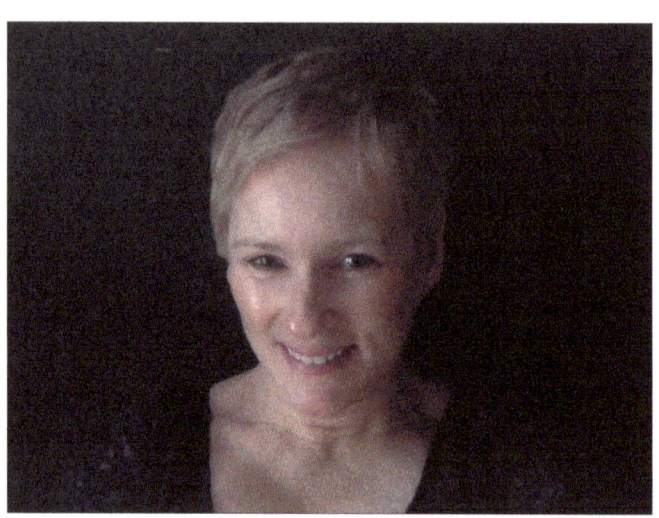

Evelin Ledebuhr

In 1970 I had my first child. He died just after birth, and I almost died too. To keep me alive, the doctor ordered a blood transfusion. With that transfusion came an unknown disease, Hepatitis C.

During the late 1970s, I started having digestive problems and developed three ulcers. My primary physician was suggesting a bland diet with dairy for the ulcers. I had recently learned that with time this treatment actually made ulcers worse. I found a physician who had an excellent nutritionist/biochemist. It took care of the ulcers, but I continued to get sicker. I developed gallbladder problems. We took care of the gall bladder, with a gallbladder cleanse that included a routine of apple juice and a beet salad with lemon and extra virgin cold pressed olive oil. My gallbladder healed, but I was still getting sicker.

I developed arthritis, fibromyalgia, lots of food allergies, and then I was misdiagnosed with systemic lupus. I changed our diet several times, eliminating sugar, white flour, and modified corn starch. After testing for allergies, I eliminated all of the problem foods for a year, then added them back one at a time to see what the affect was from each food. With all this, my health was still going downhill. I was in constant pain. For years, it hurt to be touched.

I was blessed in that I could not take most medication, due to the modified food starch binder in the meds. Modified food starch dramatically slowed my brain's processing time. If I was walking down a sidewalk talking with someone, not paying attention to what was ahead of me, and saw a street post about ten feet ahead, I couldn't process it quickly enough not to run into it. It also affected my ability to do math and remember names. This made for some embarrassing moments, until I found the cause.

Most of the prescribed medications forced me to look for natural remedies.

My nutritionist put me on supplements, but they didn't help either. What did help was the advice I got from Ann Wigmore, who advised a raw food diet and a colon cleansing. I ordered her book, *Be Your Own Doctor*, but I found it difficult to implement the concepts and guidelines. I needed coaching to be held accountable and to be away from temptation as I began this dramatic lifestyle change to a raw food diet, daily exercise, regular massages, saunas, and parasite cleanses. I went to Hippocrates Health Institute and started my journey back to health.

Within six weeks of completing the Health Educators Course, I was pain free. I regained my flexibility and strength. Most of all, I learned how an anti-inflammatory diet could begin healing my body. This information helped me to help others. I have started my own health coaching business where I combine the things that have helped me return to health.

I never made much money because I wanted more for my clients than they wanted for themselves, so I would undercharge. I had several "money mirror" issues. Also, I did know how to motivate habit change in my clients, or to instill a sense of value for what I had to offer. I did lots of continuing education, but never increased my rates as I increased my skill level in several healing modalities.

In 2006, I had a car accident that led to a long recuperation; consequently, I was not able to stay in business. I had lots of time. Since I had never read the Bible, I decided it was time. I learned that instead of turning to Elohim/God after all else fails, He asks us all to "lean not on your own understanding, in all your ways acknowledge Him, and He shall direct your paths" (Proverbs 3:5-6).

When I could return to business, I thought it wise to first learn how to do business better. This led to looking into training in how to be a health coach, while getting coaching for myself.

Through this training I met Joyce Hack, the co-editor of this book. I'm sure Joyce is a real inspiration to all who know her.

I hope my story helps you know that we are wonderfully made by our Creator, with the ability to heal when nourished properly with real, whole, raw food. Although positive results can be experienced very quickly, deep healing may take time and sometimes you need someone to coach you through it. Not only can our bodies be healed, but most importantly our thinking must change. We must be open to the help God sends to us.

> **For I know the plans I have for you, declares the LORD, plans to prosper you and not to harm you, plans to give you hope and a future.**

Jeremiah 29:11

Evelin Ledebuhr

Certified Health Coach
Bath, Michigan
evelin.ledebuhr@gmail.com

PECAN PATE' STUFFED PEPPERS

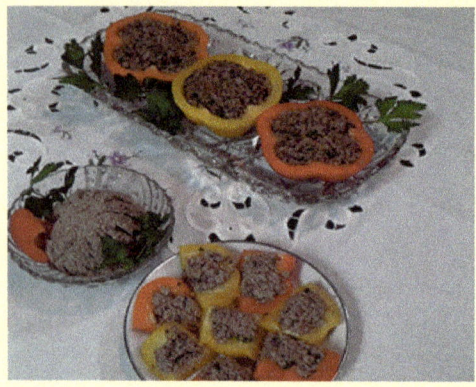

Calories	290
Protein	4g
CHO	10g
Fat	26g
Sugar	3g
Sodium	55mg
Fiber	5g
Chol	0mg

Serves 6   Per serving

INGREDIENTS

- 2 cups raw pecans (Rinse and soak pecans for 15 to 30 minutes, then rinse again and let dry a little on a paper towel. This can be done ahead of time and stored in the refrigerator in an open container.)
- ¾ medium red onion, diced
- ½ teaspoon Bragg's liquid aminos
- ½ lemon, juiced
- 4 sprigs parsley
- 1 large red bell pepper, seeded and cut in large chunks
- 1 large yellow bell pepper, seeded and cut in large chunks

DIRECTIONS

Put all ingredients, *except* the peppers, into a food processor. Process until it looks like soaked Grape Nuts cereal. Some prefer to process more. Fill pepper chunks or boats. Serve chilled.

Chef's Notes: If you grow chives or onions, use the flowers to sprinkle on the finished dish for a beautiful and tasty touch. For optional nutrition, sprinkle in a little nori, kelp, or dulse flaked or powdered seaweed.

This plates beautifully on curly greens, with edible flowers. This recipe can be used as a dip, if blended to be a little more smooth. Cut peppers and celery into dip-size pieces. I've served this for potlucks. You can also fill celery stalks.

BURSTS OF FLAVORS SLAW

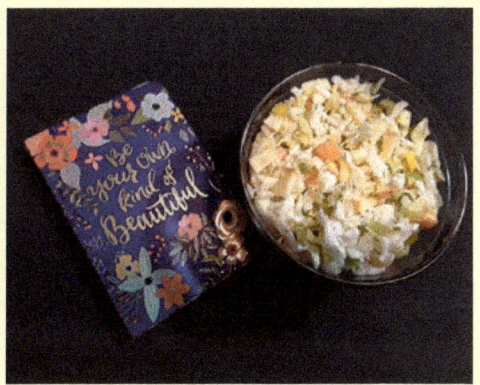

Calories	100
Protein	2g
CHO	23g
Fat	0g
Sugar	16g
Sodium	47mg
Fiber	5g
Chol	0mg

Serves 4

Per serving

INGREDIENTS

- ¼ head of cabbage
- 4 Granny Smith (or your favorite) apples
- 2 stalks celery
- 1 stalk, with leaf, bok choy (optional)
- small bulb of fennel
- 15 mint leaves (I like spearmint) Roll together and slice thinly, then slice in the opposite direction, so the pieces are very small.
- juice of 1 lime and 1 ½ navel oranges
- 1 inch of fresh ginger root, peeled and grated
- fresh grated lemon peel to taste (I grate about ¼ of the peel of an organic lemon.)

DIRECTIONS

Chop the first 5 ingredients into small pieces. (I chopped the apple right into the juice so it wouldn't turn brown.) Then mix well with juice. Grate in ginger and lemon peel and toss the salad again.

THE NUT DOESN'T FALL FAR FROM THE TREE

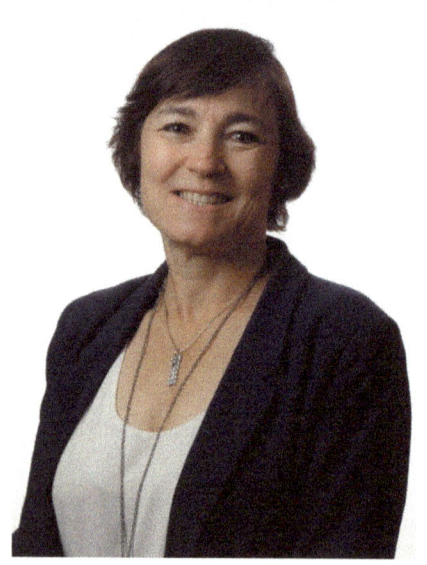

Shawnya Michaels

I grew up in Southern California. My mom was considered a bit of a health nut, and there was never any soda, typical junk food, or sugary cereals in our household. She would make cookies, only using whole wheat flour, and usually with honey instead of sugar. Breakfast would be home-ground meat patties with a fried egg or sliced bananas with plain yogurt and wheat germ.

What was considered healthy nutrition back then is a bit different than what I consider healthy today. But my education into healthy eating was started at an early age. Like all kids who feel their families are a bit different, I would cherish the opportunity to visit friends' homes where there may be a cupboard with Twinkies, Nacho Cheese Doritos, and Mystic Mint cookies!

But once I decided to become a mom myself, my upbringing kicked in, and nutritious homemade meals became a top priority. Still, what I considered healthy eating for my kids when they were young has also changed.

My eating habits and nutrition are still evolving. Nutrition science is dynamic, so some of the rules seem to change, but my lifestyle is to choose quality over quantity and focus on eating fresh, real foods.

Living in my best health means not just eating healthy, but living every day with passion and reason, keeping strong connections with friends and family, reaching out to help others in need, and developing a connection to something greater than myself.

The decision that has probably made the biggest impact on my health is to take some time every day to focus on myself. It may sound odd, but I think many women can relate to spending years so focused on family and careers that they lose sight of themselves. So making a conscious decision to take time every day to do something for myself is really what keeps my health compass pointing in the right direction.

The most recent turning point on my journey to find optimal and yummy nutrition was my husband's diagnosis with celiac disease. I was already on a low carb diet and now my husband had to make a major transformation by removing foods with gluten from his diet.

Professionally, I have been in cancer research for most of my career, and I have been obsessed with avoiding a cancer diagnosis that every other member of my immediate biological family has experienced. I have come to realize avoiding cancer may be as much about controlling stress, exercising, sleep, hydration, and eliminating toxins as it is about having optimal nutrition, and my newest passion to share all this information has led me to a new career in health coaching.

What I hope to inspire in my clients is that chronic diseases and cancer are not bad luck caused by our genes; how we live and eat influences what genes are expressed, and we do have the power to heal ourselves by changing our lifestyles.

> *It's no coincidence that four of the six letters in health are 'heal.'*
>
> **Ed Northstrum**

Shawnya Michaels, MS, MBA

Certified Health Coach
Certified Personal Trainer
El Granada, California
www.shawnyamichaels.com

EASY HOT & SOUR SOUP

One of my all-time favorite recipes is Easy Hot & Sour Soup. This is perfect for when you feel a bit under the weather, as it is a version of chicken soup, but with the extra immune boosting benefits of shiitake mushrooms, garlic, onions, and vinegar. Also, it is supper yummy! Since it is so high in protein, it is also perfect as a hearty lunch that can keep you feeling full until dinner. To up-level it, you can even make your own bone broth.

Calories	110
Protein	6g
CHO	2g
Fat	5g
Sugar	0g
Sodium	75mg
Fiber	<1g
Chol	9mg

Serves 4

Per serving

INGREDIENTS

- 4 cups low sodium chicken stock or broth
- 3 tablespoons Tamari (gluten-free) soy sauce
- ½ cup cooked organic free-range chicken, shredded
- ½ cup shiitake mushrooms, diced
- ½ tablespoon garlic chili sauce
- ¼ teaspoon ground white or black pepper
- ¼ cup white vinegar
- ⅓ cup canned bamboo shoots, julienned
- 2 tablespoons cornstarch
- 2 tablespoons cold water
- 2 green onion stalks, diced (including tops)
- ½ teaspoon toasted sesame oil

DIRECTIONS

Bring chicken broth to a simmer in a 2-quart saucepan.

Add Tamari sauce, shredded meat, mushrooms and garlic red chili sauce.

Simmer for five minutes.

Add pepper, white vinegar & bamboo shoots.

Simmer for five minutes.

Combine two tablespoons of cornstarch with two tablespoons of cold water in a cup. Stir until mixture is smooth. Add cornstarch mixture to soup and stir well.

Simmer for five minutes until soup is thickened.

Add green onions and sesame oil to soup. Stir well. Remove from heat. Serve hot.

BROWNIE ENERGY BITES

I like to keep sweets to a minimum, but pairing a cup of tea in the afternoon with an energy bite, that tastes a bit like a brownie, is a nice treat to celebrate a morning of productivity. This recipe uses maple syrup for the sweetener, which at least has a lot more nutrition in it than standard sugar. And with the protein and healthy fats from the almond butter, you can keep your metabolism on the right track!

Calories	105
Protein	4g
CHO	8g
Fat	7g
Sugar	5g
Sodium	68mg
Fiber	2g
Chol	31mg

Makes 12 bites

Per serving

INGREDIENTS

- ½ cup mashed sweet potatoes
- 2 eggs
- ¼ cup maple syrup
- ½ cup almond butter
- 1 tablespoon cocoa
- ½ teaspoon baking soda
- ½ teaspoon pumpkin pie spice or cinnamon
- 1 teaspoon vanilla extract
- ¼ cup chopped walnuts (optional)

DIRECTIONS

Place all ingredients, except the nuts, in a small food processor or bullet blender, and blend until smooth. Then add the nuts. They can be mixed in or just sprinkled on top. Spoon the batter into a greased mini muffin pan. Bake at 350°F for 15–20 minutes.

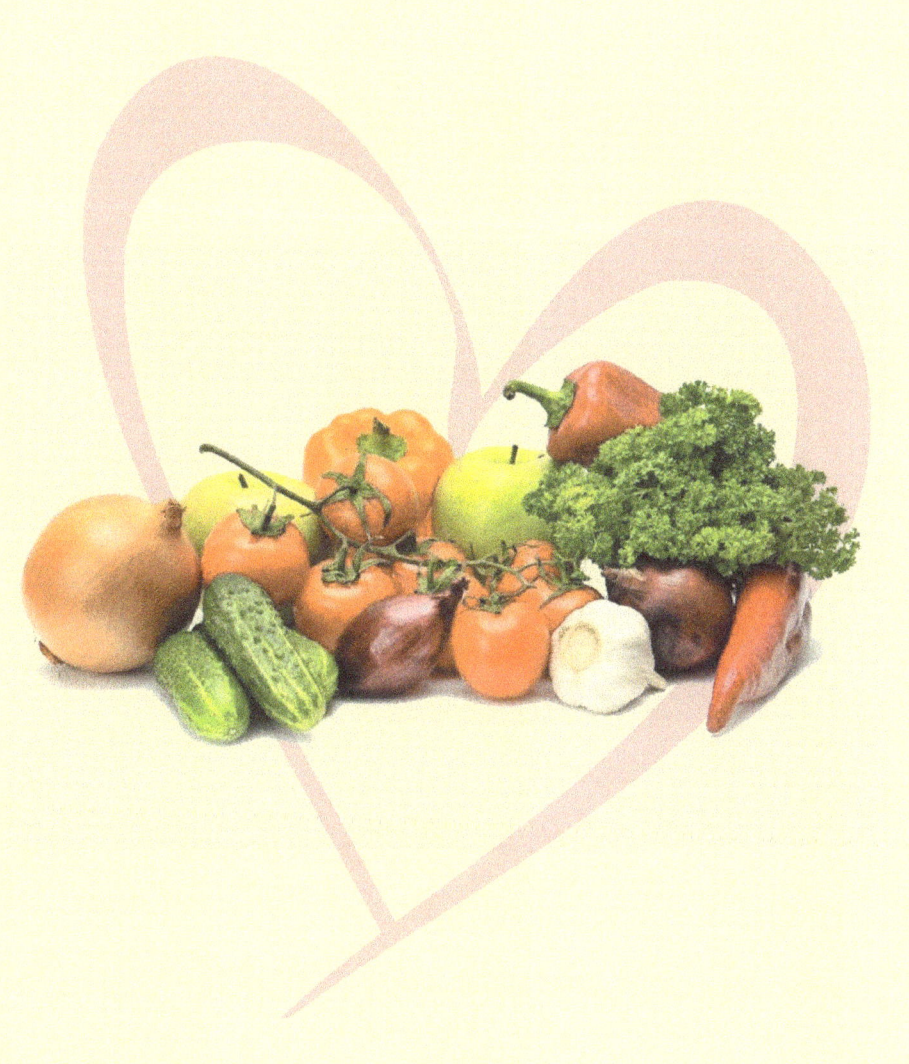

REACHING MY IDEAL WEIGHT

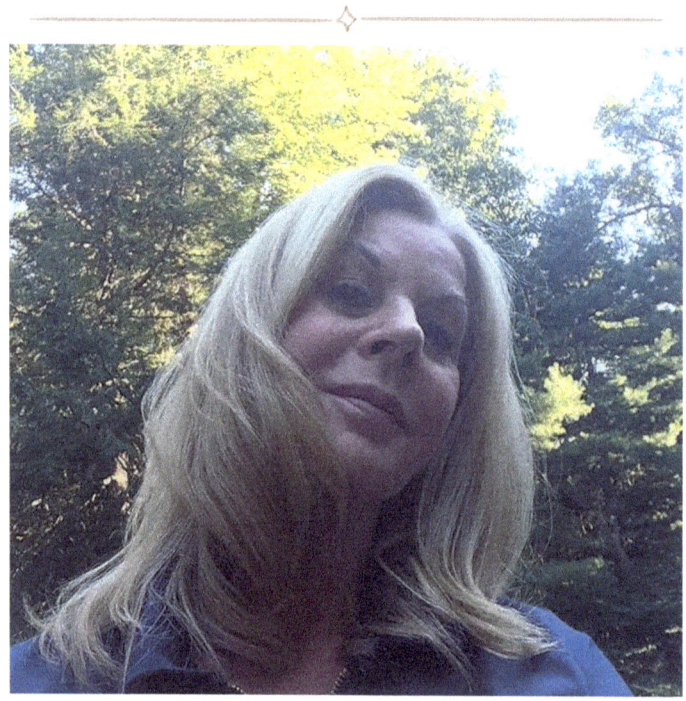

Robin Moon

Through sickness and health, here is my life story as it has played out so far. And I hope it's far from over!

Born in 1952 in the New England area to a blue-collar dad and mom, life was considered good. My parents had just purchased their first home and decided to have me come along. My twin brother and sister were twelve years old at the time. I always thought I must have been a "mistake," but I found out I was carefully planned and happily awaited. Sounds really good, right? In most ways it was good, but in terms of health it might have been better if we were a bit more wanting. Abundant times brought abundant "good" things to eat. Having lived through the depression, my parents were now merrily living the modern life. Lots of TV dinners, chocolate milk, and Wonder Bread, which was considered, at the time, to be packed with nutrients for growing kids. By the time I went to kindergarten, I was roley-poley. By third grade, we were shopping in the "Chubette" section of department stores for my clothes. Kids at school called me "fatty," my grandparents called me "healthy." Having gone through the depression, nobody wanted to be skinny. It was obvious I was my family's sign of affluence.

Reaching puberty and lusting for boys caused me to starve myself. I dropped weight and, in retrospect, I was hot! Sadly, I never saw myself in this way. Instead I was an introvert, always feeling inadequate. In my own mind I was fat, no matter what the scale or mirror told me.

Skip to age twenty-four and my first pregnancy. With sixty pounds gained, I was a walrus. My baby was wonderful and life was good, so I kept on eating with my "pregnancy" appetite. I had become a secret eater. I had a passion for donuts and coffee every afternoon, in my car and alone. When my baby turned five, I felt so ashamed as the mother, being so tired all the time; I knew I had to do something about my health. Weight Watchers! I went to the meetings with my best friend. It worked. I got down to my target weight and stayed there. Why was I so hungry? Oops, I found myself pregnant with twins.

My past habits and cravings kicked in, and this time I gained seventy pounds. The boys were born. Dealing with twins is a very adequate reason to eat anything and everything that will give you an energy spike and an endorphin boost. Yup, back to the sweets and secret eating. This time it took me almost ten years to get the weight off. I was so tired I had to sleep every afternoon before the kids came home from school just to be able to make it through dinner. I read a book called *The Endocrine Control Diet* and it changed everything. It wasn't my fault. My hormones were causing my whole system to be off. I could cure my problem with the same thing that was causing my misery—food. I went to the doctor who had written the book, and he did blood work. My results showed that I was one small step away from diabetes. That got my attention. I followed his advice, and I have never looked back. Being unhealthy was the catalyst to my paradigm shift. I had to find the diet that was just right for me. I found it and I've stuck to it for the last twenty-three years. Up and down only five or so pounds. Energy stable, health stable.

I have tried so hard to help others onto this eating regime. For the most part, I have had no luck.

More change came into my life. I had to deal with my divorce, but then I was reunited with the love of my life from over forty years ago. Moving to a new state and a new home, I decided to also recreate my career. I wanted to help people find their way to health. This new time in my life was a good time to break into a career that had real meaning.

My true passion to help people have the health and vitality I have sought so long and hard to capture sealed my decision to get training. Health Coach Institute came along, and I grabbed at the chance to train as a health coach. The training solidified all my research on health and wellness and gave me a whole new arsenal to work with. Now I understand that each and every person must find their unique diet, as well as when, what, and how to eat for their own body and life.

It is such a thrill to help people navigate this rolling river of choices. In the end, it is so easy … once you know how! I have endless empathy for those who either don't have the information to create the best health for themselves or those who simply can't overcome the obstacles without support. If there is anything I can share with others that might inspire them to eat a healthier more nutritious diet, I would remind them that "Health Really Is Their Only Wealth." As we age, we have so much wisdom. So much to share with the world. What a shame if we are too tired or too sick to share all that we have to give. I believe that God has placed every remedy for every ill right at our fingertips. It is for us to discover what those individual remedies are for ourselves. The first step is to eat a healthy diet and stop throwing roadblocks to our own health in the way with the less-than-healthy foods we ingest. When our time comes, will we wish we had only had more junk foods? Or will we wish that we had heeded our better judgement about what would give us active longevity?

> Seek to live with the Truth as only the Truth will set you free.

L. Ron Hubbard

Robin Moon

Certified Health Coach
Certified Life Coach
Personal Fitness Trainer
RobinsHealthyTransformations@gmail.com

BLUEBERRY PANCAKES

Delicious blueberries mixed in with the light flavor and airy texture of coconut flour will make this recipe your new favorite! These blueberry pancakes are free from wheat and other grains, and have a low score on the glycemic index with almond flour and coconut flour. No more box pancake mixes for your family!

Makes 2 servings

Calories	292
Protein	19g
CHO	16g
Fat	17g
Sugar	9g
Sodium	327mg
Fiber	4g
Chol	93mg

Per serving

INGREDIENTS

- 1 cup almond flour
- 1 tablespoon coconut flour, finely ground
- 1 teaspoon baking powder
- pinch of salt
- 2 egg whites
- 1 egg
- ¼ cup non-dairy milk
- 4 drops liquid stevia
- 1 teaspoon vanilla extract
- ⅓ cup fresh blueberries
- 1 tablespoon olive oil, for greasing

FOR TOPPING

- ½ cup fresh blueberries

DIRECTIONS

In a medium bowl, combine the almond flour, coconut flour, salt and baking powder. Set aside.

Place the eggs, stevia drops, vanilla and milk in a small bowl and whisk well.

Add egg mixture to dry ingredients, whisk until just combined, do not overmix. Gently stir in the blueberries.

Preheat a large pan over medium heat. Lightly grease the pan with olive oil.

For each pancake, spoon ¼ cup of the pancake mixture onto pan. Cook until surface of pancakes have some bubbles and sides of the pancake firm up, about 2–3 minutes.

Carefully flip the pancakes with a thin spatula, and cook the underside, for another 45 seconds. Continue with remaining mixture.

Serve the pancakes warm, topped with fresh blueberries.

FRUIT SOUP

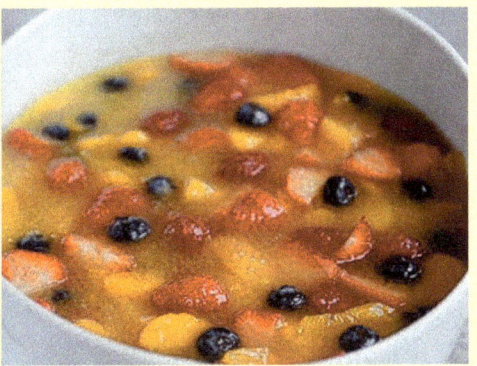

Calories	136
Protein	1g
CHO	34g
Fat	0g
Sugar	23g
Sodium	11mg
Fiber	1g
Chol	0mg

Serves 16

Per serving

INGREDIENTS

- 3 ½ cups pineapple juice, unsweetened
- 1 ½ cups grapes, seedless, sliced
- 3 bananas, sliced
- 3 ½ tablespoons minute tapioca
- 2 (29 ounce) cans peaches, diced
- 3 cups strawberries or raspberries, sliced
- mint leaf, for garnish

DIRECTIONS

Soak tapioca for 5 minutes in pineapple juice.

Cook juice and tapioca on medium until thick, stirring continuously.

Add fruits to thickened sauce.

Serve warm, or better yet, chill!

Garnish with fresh sliced banana and a mint leaf.

MY JOURNEY TO HOLISTIC HEALTH COACH

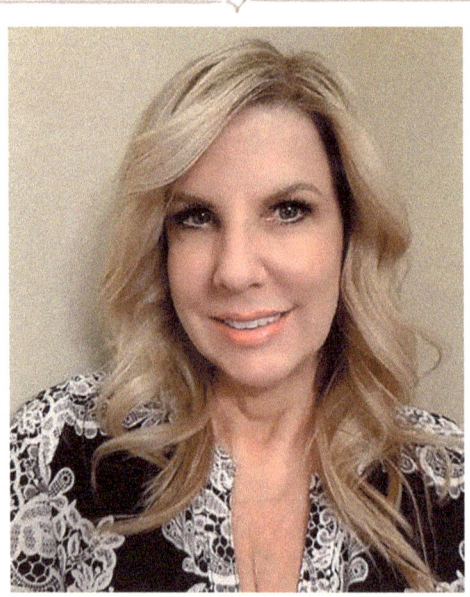

Charleen Cuellar

Growing up in Covina, California, in a middle-class family, we ate the normal American diet: hamburgers, pork chops, steak, chicken, hot dogs, liver, mashed potatoes, fries, peas, corn on the cob, Italian food, cold and hot sugar laden cereals, sodas, milk, and concentrated orange juice. As an active child, I participated in lots of activities, such as riding my bike, skating, and walking around the neighborhood with my friends, siblings, my aunt and cousins. Although I was not in any organized sports, I wanted to learn martial arts. My family could not afford the cost of tuition, so I practiced with my cousins. I also did

Tae Kwon Do for a couple of years when I was in my thirties. I have continued to be active well into my forties: swimming, working out, lifting weights, circuit training, cardio, Pilates, and taking long walks.

My dear Italian grandmother (Ma) was passionate about health. She emphasized that eating wholesome foods, exercising, drinking good water, and being positive and optimistic was important. She taught me to look at the world with a smile and to be a friendly person. She also taught me to be cautious and have eyes all around my head, as it's better to be safe than sorry. She taught me about processed foods, how they were laden with chemicals and preservatives, and their adverse affect on our health; she also taught me how to read food labels. I remember her taking me to the health food store and enjoying the many options available. One experience I really enjoyed was exercising with her to Jack LaLanne on TV. We took long walks together, and she would say, "Let's go window shopping!" So we took long walks along the sidewalk past many stores and would look at all the pretty things in the windows. She taught me about keeping good posture while sitting and walking, and she always said, "Onion is king and garlic is queen. They are God's natural antibiotics and laughter is the best medicine of all." Ma lived to be ninety-seven years old! I am so grateful and will always cherish all the wisdom she has shared with me throughout the years. What Ma has taught me has been a beacon to my calling of health coaching.

Needless to say, with all that my Ma has taught me, I am and have always been passionate about health and wellness. Throughout the years knowing my passion for health and helping others, my family and friends have come to me for help, and I would go on a mission to help them and loved doing so. I have done research ever since I can remember on health, foods, exercise, anything to do with health and wellness.

So how did I become so sick and then end up with my new career/calling into health coaching? Where to start. Well, I got married at nineteen, but it didn't work out and I became a single mom for many years. Being a mom and a grandma is one of the best things that has ever happened to me, and I am so blessed by each one of my three grown children and two grandsons.

Throughout the years, I have had many stressful times. I was the sole provider of my family for a very long time, and money was tight. I did the best I could with feeding my children and myself. But we had times where I could not afford to buy nutritious foods, and we had to resort to eating cheap packaged and canned foods. It goes now without saying that we are either going to pay at the grocery store, or pay with our health, quality of life, medical bills, and finances.

In my early forties I remarried and moved from San Clemente, California, where I absolutely loved living because of the beauty and the weather, to Kalispell, Montana, because of my husband's military transfer. I had experienced many life changes which caused stress, and my weight started to climb. I lost my energy, had major stomach problems, became depressed, and had anxiety, high cholesterol, insomnia, and more.

Gradually, we drifted more and more to eating fast foods. Most of the time, I would pick the healthiest food on the menu, but I drank diet soda quite a bit. Eating fast food and drinking diet soda only made things worse; I just didn't feel well anymore and ended up losing my gallbladder. My doctors kept giving me meds to help my symptoms, and if I had taken every medication I was prescribed, I would be a walking medicine chest.. I'm not advocating that you don't take your prescribed meds; I just didn't want to be on so much medication because I knew I could help myself in holistic ways to heal. I didn't want to put a Band-aid on my symptoms; I wanted it to be my personal choice.

I decided to go on a journey to heal myself. I have changed my eating habits, and I stopped drinking Diet Coke. (I don't drink any soda.) I drink lots of water, eat whole, organic foods as much as possible, and move my body in ways I find enjoyable and not painful. I found a functional doctor, found out what all of the illnesses I had developed over time were, and so far I have been able to get myself off medications for my stomach and high cholesterol, which I have been taking for many years. I still have a ways to go on this journey.

After having to give up my beauty business and being told that I should go on disability, I did not want to give up and stop working. I was determined to find something that I could do from home that didn't cause me pain. As I searched, I knew that I wanted to work in the health and wellness field, as this is what I love and am very passionate about. Some things I considered were becoming an acupuncturist, naturopathic doctor, or herbalist. I said a prayer, then I went back to my computer and opened up my email account, and there was an ad for becoming a health coach. I had never heard of a health coach before. I instantly knew this was my path! I was actually already doing this for many years to help family and friends who had health issues.

I attended and graduated as a health coach from the Institute for Integrative Nutrition, and now I am finishing up my training at the Health Coach Institute as a certified health coach!

There are too many people today who are sick due to eating processed foods that are laden with chemicals and foods that are not right for their own bodies; they are stressed, have toxins in their environments, and are living a sedentary lifestyle. I have had too many family members and friends who have had cancer, diabetes, obesity, arthritis, heart disease, and many other illnesses and diseases.

My mission is to help others to live well in all areas of their lives, to help them discover what foods are best for their body and how to relieve stress, be healthy, and stay that way through my methods of health coaching. I want to spread the word about eating whole, nutritious foods and share the message of how eating clean can benefit our lives, as well as how eating the wrong foods for our bodies, and foods laden with chemicals, can make us very sick, take away our quality of life, be a financial strain, and even shorten our lives. I want to help as many people as I can to live long, happy, healthy, fulfilled lives.

My recommendations to the world would be to make your health a priority. Eat whole, nutritious foods. Drink lots of filtered water. Find activities that you love and get outside in the sun. Spend time with family and friends. Smile, laugh, be positive, have goals and aspirations. By doing this, you can live a life full of good health, happiness, love, and wonder.

Eat for good health so you can live your best life!

> Let food be thy medicine and
> medicine be thy food.

Hippocrates

Charleen Cuellar

Holistic Health & Wellness Coach
Murrieta, California
charleencuellar@gmail.com
www.wellnesstransformationscoach.com

HEALTHY VEGGIE OMELET

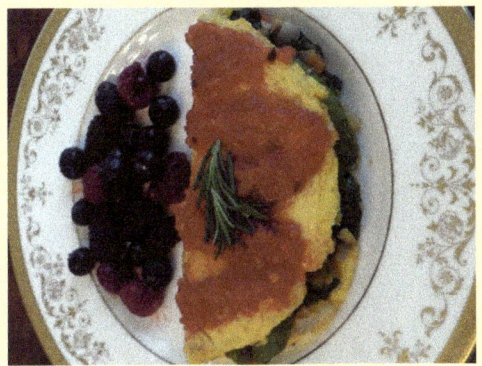

Calories	461
Protein	24g
CHO	17g
Fat	20g
Sugar	9g
Sodium	300mg
Fiber	9g
Chol	0mg

Makes one omelet   Per recipe

INGREDIENTS

- 1 teaspoon olive oil
- 1 cup pre-washed organic baby spinach
- ½ small organic tomato, diced
- ¼ cup organic onion, diced
- 3 organic egg whites
- pinch of Himalayan sea salt & pepper, to taste
- ½ small organic avocado, sliced
- organic salsa of choice
- fresh berries, for side

DIRECTIONS

In a small nonstick frying pan add the olive oil, turn on heat to medium/low, then add the onion, tomato and spinach. Mix and sauté about 3 minutes until done and set aside on a small plate.

Scramble the egg whites in a bowl with a fork; add the salt and pepper to taste and pour into the same frying pan that you used to sauté the veggies. As the egg whites start to cook, gently push the sides in with a spatula and tilt pan to allow the uncooked egg white to run into the pan to cook. When egg white is almost all cooked and stable enough, flip over and cook the other side.

Add the cooked veggies onto the front half of the omelette, add sliced avocado on top of cooked veggies, and fold the other half of the omelette over the veggies. Transfer to plate and top with salsa to taste. Add a side of fresh berries or other fruit and enjoy!

HEARTY SPICY ORGANIC CHICKEN VEGGIE SOUP

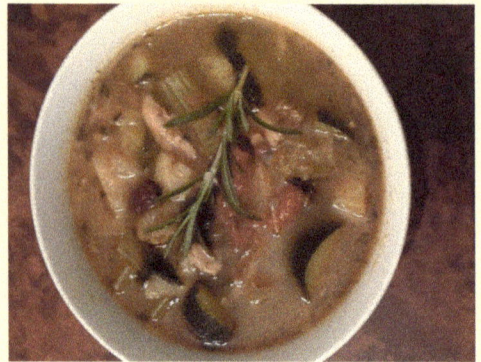

Calories	253
Protein	33g
CHO	21g
Fat	3g
Sugar	6g
Sodium	283mg
Fiber	8g
Chol	0mg

Serves 12

Per serving

INGREDIENTS

- 4 pounds whole organic free-range chicken
- 3 boxes organic low sodium chicken broth (32 fluid ounce boxes)
- 1 organic onion or leek, chopped
- 5 organic celery stocks, sliced into chunks
- 5 cloves organic garlic, minced
- 1 whole bay leaf
- 2 peppercorns
- 2 cloves
- 3 tablespoons poultry seasoning
- ¼–½ teaspoon ground cayenne pepper
- 1 sprig fresh rosemary or ½ teaspoon dried rosemary
- ¼ teaspoon of turmeric
- pinch of Himalayan salt
- ½ head organic green cabbage, chopped
- 1 (28 ounce) can organic kidney beans, drained
- 4 organic zucchini squash, chopped
- 1 small (8 ounce) package organic frozen cut up broccoli or two stalks cut into florets
- 1 (28 ounce) can Muir Glen organic fire roasted diced tomatoes
- 1 bunch organic kale, stems cut off and discarded, chopped

DIRECTIONS

Rinse and place whole chicken into a large pot. Pour in the 3 boxes of chicken broth, add the chopped onion, celery, minced garlic, bay leaf, peppercorns, cloves, poultry seasoning, ground cayenne pepper, rosemary, turmeric and Himalayan salt. Bring to a boil, then cover and simmer until chicken is done, about 1½ to 2 hours. Carefully remove chicken and place on large plate or cutting board, remove the meat, and chop into pieces, discarding the bones.

Add the cabbage, kidney beans, zucchini, broccoli, diced tomatoes, and the cooked chicken chunks to the broth. Cover and bring back to a boil and simmer on medium low heat for about 10 minutes, until the zucchini and cabbage is almost done. Add the kale and cook for a couple minutes longer so the kale is cooked but not overdone.

Remove from heat and serve. Top with a sprinkle of crushed pink Himalayan salt.

For leftover soup, just heat up what you will be using in a smaller pot so that you won't be overcooking the veggies each time you reheat them. Do not heat in the microwave, as this will deplete all the nutrients.

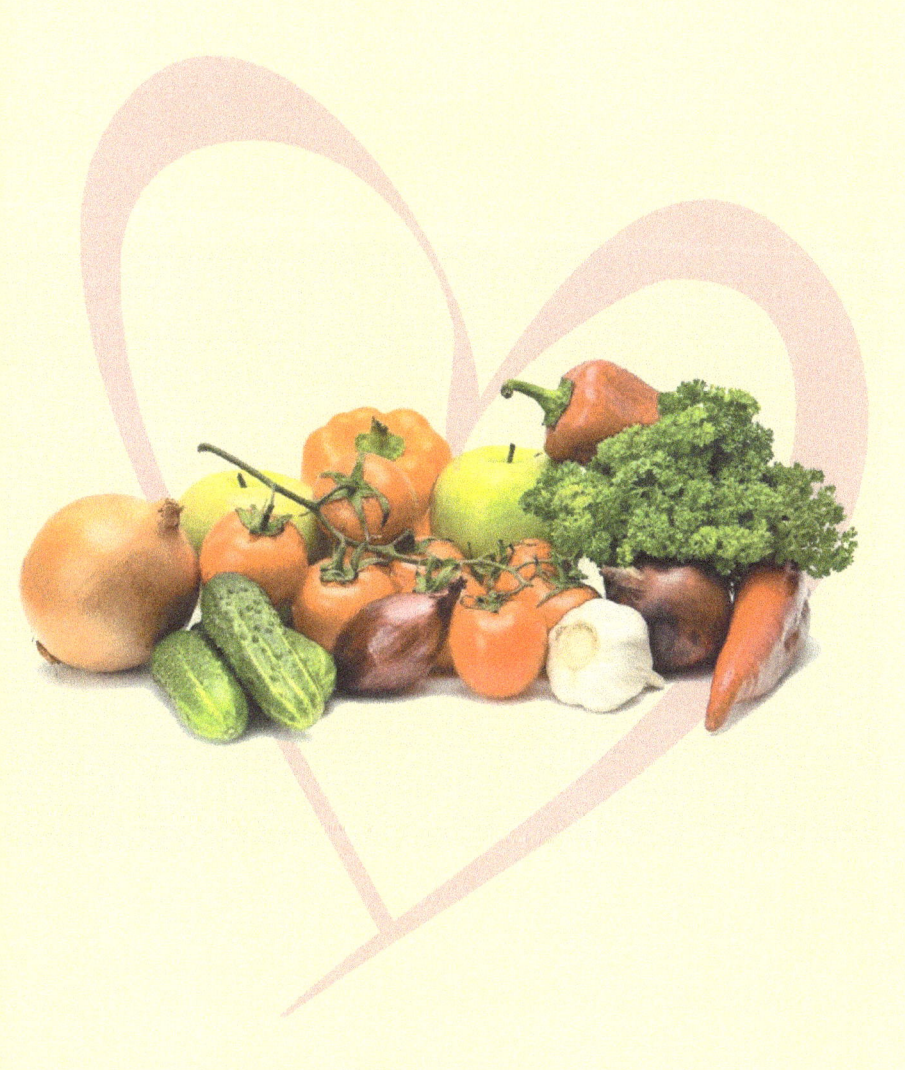

MAKE CHANGES NOW— DON'T WAIT

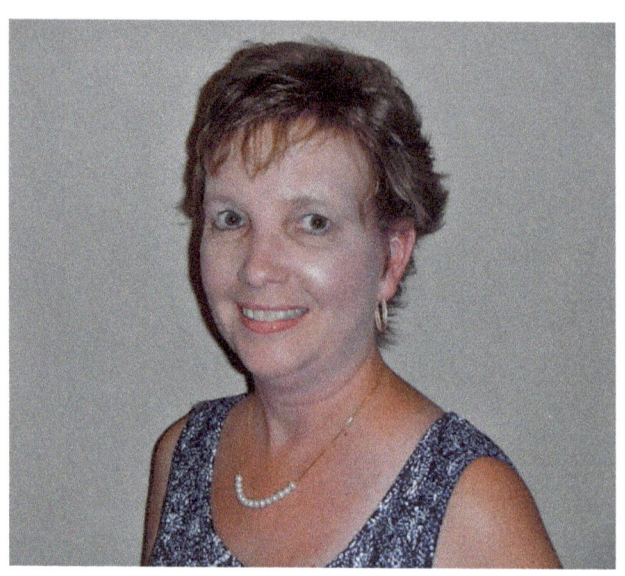

Peggy Heaton

I grew up in Cincinnati, Ohio, and lived with my parents in a small town called Norwood, Ohio. I was the baby of the family with four amazing older sisters. On occasion, my sisters became jealous because my parents showed special attention to me, as it seemed that I was often getting my own way.

My parents were the best parents ever. They taught us first that faith was what will get us through, no matter what challenges we face. They taught and demonstrated principles that are still part of my life today, which include values and morals, but the most important was how to love unconditionally. One of mom's favorite sayings when things got tough was, "This too shall pass." My loving parents passed onto a better life in 2008 and left a legacy for my sisters and I that gave us the courage and strength to face any challenge in life. They always live on in our hearts.

Growing up, healthy eating wasn't a regular conversation in our home. My father was a fire fighter, and his favorite breakfast was eggs and bacon. He was always known for his strength and heroism in saving lives. As a family, we ate well, however we depended upon the more traditional meals, like meat and potatoes. Vegetables were part of every meal, but dad always had to have his chocolate chip cookies or some sweet treat after every meal. It was his way of telling his stomach, "I'm done eating."

I wish I knew then what I know now about eating because it is more difficult to give up sweets now. At this time, eating the way we did had no effect on my weight. I was thin all the way through high school and really didn't pay too much attention to what I ate, which included bread, cookies, and soft drinks. It really wasn't until I hit menopause that I began to gain weight, which had a major effect on me. My sleep changed, my weight was out of control, and I felt like a hot mess.

I started to feel like something was missing in my life but wasn't sure what it was. I struggled with who I wanted to be when I grew up and started to take a look at some of my interests; one of those was the health field. I had considered becoming a health coach, but to be honest I was afraid that I didn't have what was required and not sure if I could overcome the challenges. When my husband's office closed its doors in 2016, that was the time for me to step up and do something. In March of 2016, I made a decision to register with Health Coach Institute and become a health coach. I can't tell you how happy I am for taking that step and how this program has changed my life.

I have learned to eat healthier and have developed strategies that have increased my belief in *me* and in knowing what it takes to succeed in all areas of my life. As a mother, I have many things to be grateful for, including my two wonderful sons. Although challenges show up in our lives, it is how we handle the challenges that make the difference. When my youngest son was diagnosed as being on the autism spectrum, I was not sure how to handle the situation. However, we have managed to learn, grow, and make the best of it; although, the stress that I encounter on some days is that of a combat soldier.

My food regimen consists of eating more greens, plus fruits and vegetables. This has helped to keep both my weight and stress level in check. I have also incorporated more exercise into my life and some days I feel like I'm at the top of the world. I think I've become more aware of what I need to be doing, and deciding to eat healthy is something that would be helpful for everyone. You can't force good nutrition on anyone, but you can share the knowledge that you have that will make others' lives better. I opened my heart and mind to eating healthy and moving more, which has helped me to pay attention to my needs and what makes me feel good. As I make space for self-care for myself, I can teach others how to do the same.

My final words are to encourage everyone to take action. Do not wait! Now is the time. Life is too short to be unhealthy and miserable. Take a good look in the mirror and pay attention to what you need as awareness is the key to taking action toward making changes in your life. When your cup is full, you can give to others more than what you think. If you want to give your very best to your friends and family, be aware of the things in your life that work well for you, then take action to move away from the things that don't serve you.

My message is, "Life is too short to be unhealthy and miserable. Don't wait, do it now."

> *When you speak from your heart and say the words your soul has only dared to whisper, that's when miracles happen.*

Peggy Heaton

Certified Health Coach
Woodstock, Georgia
www.balancedlivingnow.net
peggy@balancedlivingnow.net

SCRAMBLED TOFU

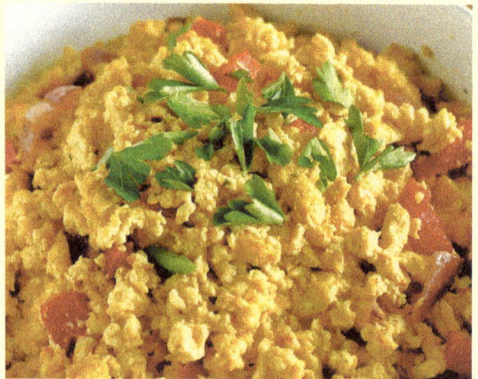

Calories	80
Protein	8g
CHO	3g
Fat	4g
Sugar	0g
Sodium	107mg
Fiber	1g
Chol	0mg

Serves 4

Per serving

INGREDIENTS

- 1 package medium/firm tofu
- ½ teaspoon garlic powder
- ½ teaspoon onion powder
- ⅛–¼ teaspoon turmeric
- ½ tablespoon dried parsley flakes
- ½ tablespoon Bragg's liquid aminos
- 2 teaspoons chicken-style seasoning
- ½ tablespoon nutritional yeast flakes
- fresh parsley, for garnish
- tomato wedges, for garnish

DIRECTIONS

Preheat a large nonstick frying pan to medium heat.

Drain and rinse tofu. Chop and mash tofu with spoon into frying pan.

Sprinkle all seasonings equally over tofu. Mix well.

Stir occasionally. Cook until most of the moisture has disappeared, approximately 10 minutes. Serve fresh and hot.

Garnish with fresh parsley and tomato wedges.

CHRISTMAS FRUITCAKE

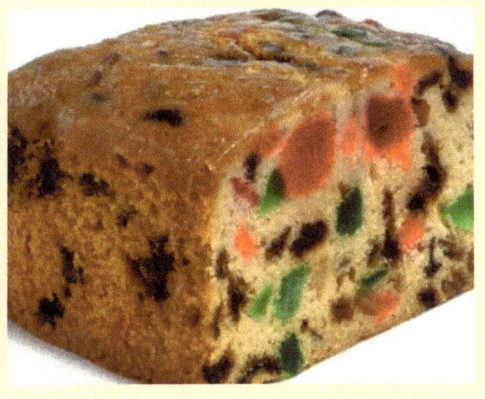

	Per serving
Calories	225
Protein	4g
CHO	41g
Fat	5g
Sugar	27g
Sodium	5mg
Fiber	4g
Chol	0mg

Serves 12

INGREDIENTS

- ¾ cup pineapple juice, unsweetened
- 1 teaspoon vanilla
- 1 cup mixed raw nuts
- 1 ½ cups mixed dried fruit
- ½ cup dates, chopped
- ½ cup cranberries, dried
- 1 cup raisins
- 1 tablespoon Ener-G egg replacer powder (available online or at any health food store, 1 egg = 1 ½ teaspoon egg replacer + 2 tablespoons water)
- ¼ cup honey
- ½ teaspoon cinnamon or substitute
- ¼ teaspoon allspice
- 1 ½ teaspoons baking powder
- 2 cups spelt flour

DIRECTIONS

Preheat oven to 350°F. Mix all ingredients together in a mixing bowl in the order given.

Pour dough into a 9-inch round or square clear glass baking dish that has been lightly greased, using a nonstick spray. Bake at 350°F for 45 minutes or until golden brown and an inserted toothpick comes out clean.

Chef's note: You may also use two small (3" x 7") loaf pans.

Life Is a Candle

Life is a candle that glows
    Night and day,
You only have one,
    So why waste it away?
It isn't a flame you can
    Light now and then,
For once it goes out
    You can't start it again.
So treasure the gift and
    Its brilliance enhance,
For health, as you know,
    Comes by choice
Not by chance!

ABOUT THE AUTHOR
"Tragedy to Triumph"

Joyce Hack

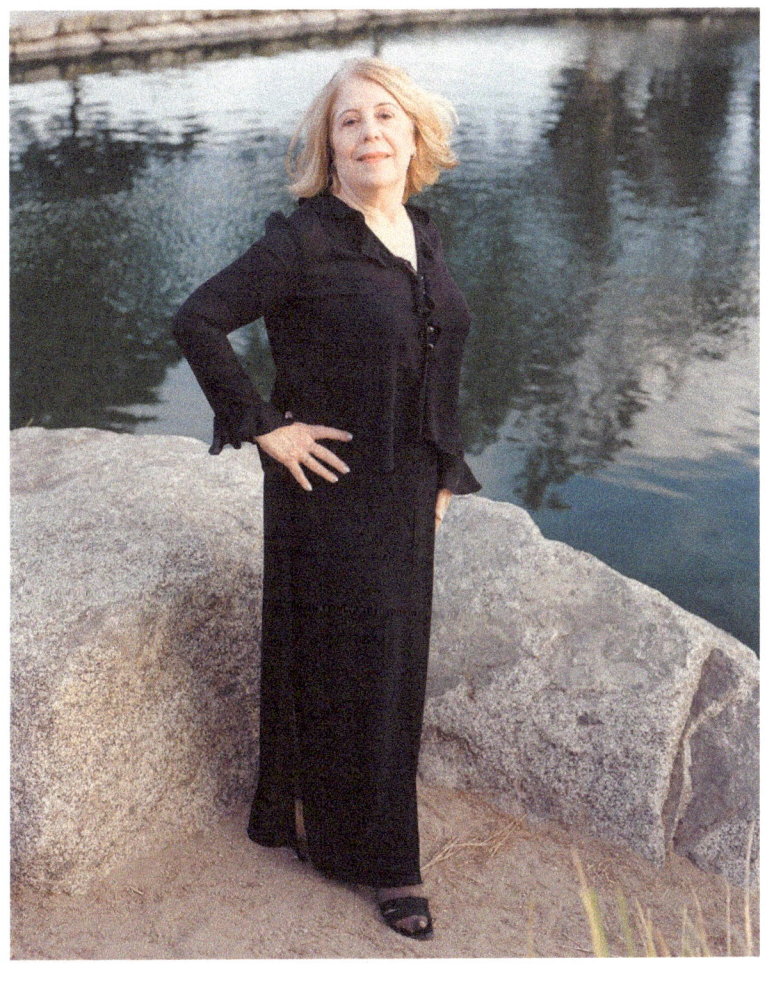

No words can describe the devastation and pain I felt when I lost my husband, soul mate, best friend, and the love of my life in a tragic accident. We had just moved to California from Canada to pursue our dreams together. With his death, I was left behind with two young daughters far from our family and friends in Canada. Much like an architect, I had to go back to the drawing board and write out plans to build a new life for my family. What I have learned is that we can turn scars into stars and tragedy into triumph. What makes the difference? It's our attitude that largely determines our altitude. It's these obstacles that challenge us with neverending opportunities to grow and to learn, to become more resilient, and to make us into better and stronger people.

My hope is that my work involves an understanding of peace as you walk your own path in life and that this peace inspires you to discover your own limitlessness. I offer a professional experience spanning more than thirty-five years in food production, clinical nutrition and management in North America.

I am a certified Health and Wellness Coach, a Registered Dietitian Nutritionist (RDN), and a nutritional consultant to heart health research programs conducted at Loma Linda University, School of Public Health. As a chef, I have trained many cooks and bakers.

Someone has called me the "secret ingredient in a recipe for inspiration." It is true; I am consistently challenging my clients to commit themselves to living their lives with purpose, action, and courage. My focus is on personal health and growth in every area of my clients' lives.

I am a mother and grandmother who loves to grow roses and celebrate their beauty. I have two precious grandchildren whom I adore. I collect antiques, host my friends and family, and through my reading I am committed to continuous self-development. I am an effective leader committed to positive outcomes in all aspects of life. I inspire others through thoughtfulness and unconditional love.

My motto is, "Love with an uninhibited soul and turn challenges into triumphs." I am looking forward to working with you in your challenges of life and assisting you in going from triumph to triumph.

Joyce Hack, RDN,

Certified Health Coach
www.feelingfabulousoverfifty.com
Joyinred@verizon.net
www.5linx.net/jhack (click on opportunity)

ABOUT THE AUTHOR
"From Health Challenges to Health Coaching"

Linda McLeod

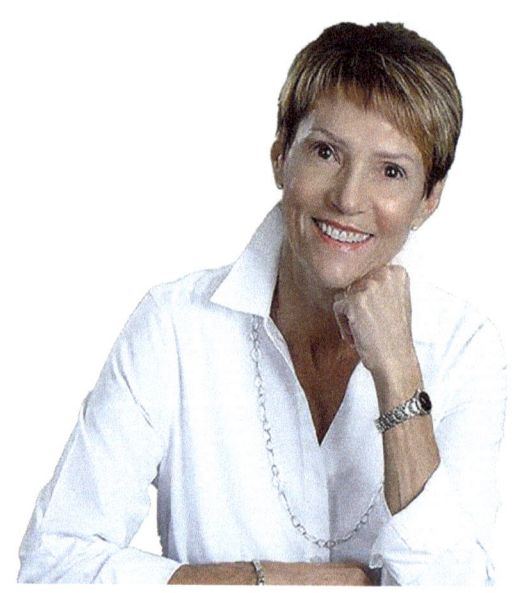

My passion and knowledge of health, and becoming a consummate health coach, emerged from wake-up calls that forced me to entrust myself to find solutions to difficult conditions.

There were my own health challenges: As a child of ten years, I missed an entire year of school because of my hepatitis, a serious liver condition that only resolved itself over time. My family began to rely increasingly on healthy, whole foods, or foods-as-grown, simply prepared without too much sugar, salt, and fat. A few years later, now working for a large corporation involving extensive travel and a hectic work schedule and being on my own, a major health challenge turned into a hospitalization of three months. This brought me back once more to the natural diet of my younger years. And yet, I only learned my lessons slowly. The next health crisis almost cost me my life. With my good dietary practices shot, a common-place pneumonia—not properly treated for two years by my physicians—developed into a very serious lung condition. With little hope for recovery, the best my pulmonary specialist doctor could recommend was a lifetime of antibiotics. This was my major wake-up call. I realized I had to get more serious about becoming a better prepared medical consumer and to learn all I could about the body's ability to heal itself—if treated well with a health-compatible lifestyle.

But then I also had a health crisis centering on a member of my family. The life of my sixteen-year-old son, being the oldest and having been without a father for some time, was demonstrating some difficult behavior. Eventually being diagnosed with ADHD (Attention-Deficit Hyperactivity Disorder), his treatment team strongly recommended Ritalin. Instead, I put him on a diet devoid of dairy and sugar. And his turnaround began at once. It totally changed his life: he calmed down; he became well-adjusted; he loved school and excelled.

Having weathered these crises, I began to recognize the power of therapeutic lifestyle change in turning even serious diseases around. I learned about the large body of knowledge available, filling whole floors of libraries. With my confidence in these new, more natural treatment options growing, my background in business and education, and with my passion in wanting to help women to find a more balanced and fulfilling life, it was quite natural for me to make health and wellness coaching my career.

Now I guide women through a process to discover their desires and goals that will take them on a journey to help them stop wanting things and start engaging in the process of creating them, with health at the center.

Registered with the Canadian Association for Integrative Nutrition and the Canadian Health Coach Alliance and with a degree in Organizational and Business Management, I am now at your service as your Health and Lifestyle Coach.

Linda McLeod

Certified Health and Lifestyle Coach
www.healthhabits4life.com
linda@healthhabits4life.com

RECIPE NAMES BY CO-AUTHOR

QUINOA SALAD 43
ROASTED EGGPLANT WITH KALE,
FRESH MOZZARELLA AND PINENUTS 45

- Joyce Hack

GREEN BEANS AND RED PEPPER SIDE DISH 50
WILD RICE AND APPLE STUFFED ACORN SQUASH 51

- Linda McLeod

CREAMY CARROT & GINGER SOUP 58
VEGETABLE FLAX CRACKERS 59
VANILLA ICE CREAM 60

- Theresa Nicassio

BASIC STIR-FRY 65
GENTLE LENTIL SOUP 65

- Stacey Morgenstern

THAI SQUASH STEW 69
SUPER VEGGIE SOUP 69
ROASTED SALMON WITH MANGO STRAWBERRY SALSA 70

- Carey Peters

MINT JULEP DRINK 78
SWEET POTATO BISQUE 79
CARIBBEAN MANGO SALSA 79

- Chef AJ

LOVING HEALTHY LIVING

CHARLEEN'S SULTRY SWEET CORN SOUP 84
THANKSGIVING MARVELOUS SWEET POTATO
CARROT PUREE 85

- Martha Green

DAN DAN ZOODLES 91
O-REN ISHII'S MISO SOUP 92

- Chad Curtis

HEALTHY LEFTOVER MEAL 97
BROWN RICE QUINOA PASTA WITH PESTO & FIGS 98

- Tina Jordan Amoah

CARROT CAKE 104
GRANOLA 105

-Meg Zeleny

BLACK BEAN CUPCAKES 109
HAZELNUT CREAM FROSTING 110
MIXED BERRY GINGER COMPOTE 110
ASIAN INSPIRED SALAD 111

- Samantha Schmuck

ASIAN SALMON BOWL 115
CASHEW AND PEPPER STIR FRY 116

- Bertha Noble

RAW ENERGY BARS 125
COCONUT OIL CHOCOLATE SQUARES 126

- Nicole Jennifer Enns

HEALTHY SPICED BANANA BREAD 130
VEGGIE EGG WHITE MUFFIN 131

- Brittany Johnson

FENNEL AND ORANGE SALAD 136
COCONUT BERRY AND PECAN CEREAL 137

- Hollie Ancharoff

KID APPROVED ALLERGY FRIENDLY PUMPKIN MUFFINS 142
KID APPROVED ALLERGY FREE WAFFLES 143

- Amber Anderson

BLACK BEAN AND ZUCCHINI TACOS 147
HOMEMADE BLACK BEANS 148
HOMEMADE CORN TORTILLAS 148

- Kirsten Ault

TROPICAL CHEESECAKE 154
HUMMUS 155

- Holly Kelsey

EGG WHITE FRITTATA 159
POST WORKOUT PROTEIN SHAKE 160

- Dan Ferrato

CHIA PORRIDGE 158
BEAN BURGERS 159

- Dana Camera

ITALIAN BAKED HADDOCK 166
RUSTIC MUSHROOM POLENTA 167

- Jessica Geist

TUNA AND AVOCADO SALAD 178
CHICKEN AND APPLE SANDWICH 178

- Lucie Woods

STUFFED SWEET POTATOES 183
CREAMED PEAR TOPPING 184
- **Laura Stempky**

HALIBUT SKEWERS 190
SMOKED SALMON AVOCADO BREAKFAST
WITH YOGURT & FRESH BLUEBERRIES 191
- **Donna Willon**

PECAN PATÉ STUFFED PEPPERS 196
BURST OF FLAVORS SLAW 197
- **Evelin Ledebum**

EASY HOT AND SOUR SOUP 201
BROWNIE ENERGY BITES 202
- **Shawnya Michaels**

BLUEBERRY PANCAKES 208
FRUIT SOUP 209
- **Robin Moon**

HEALTHY VEGGIE OMELET 215
HEARTY SPICY ORGANIC CHICKEN VEGGIE SOUP 216
- **Charleen Cuellar**

SCRAMBLED TOFU 222
CHRISTMAS FRUIT CAKE 223
- **Peggy Heaton**

CONVERSION CHART

The recipes featured in this book were all developed using standard US measures. The charts below offer equivalents for US and metric measures. Please keep in mind that all conversions are approximate and have been rounded up or down to the nearest whole number.

VOLUME CONVERSIONS	
US	METRIC
1 teaspoon	5 milliliters
1 tablespoon	15 milliliters
¼ cup	59 milliliters
⅓ cup	79 milliliters
½ cup	118 milliliters
1 cup	237 milliliters
1½ cups	355 milliliters
4 cups (1 quart)	.946 liter
1.06 quarts	1 liter
4 quarts (1 gallon)	3.8 liters

WEIGHT CONVERSIONS	
OUNCES	GRAMS
½	14
¾	21
1	28
1½	43
2	57
2½	71
3	85
3½	99
4	113
4½	128
5	142
10	283
12	340
16 (1 pound)	454

CPSIA information can be obtained
at www.ICGtesting.com
Printed in the USA
LVHW05s0459210418
574263LV00020B/189/P